FINAL CHOICES

AUTONOMY IN
HEALTH CARE DECISIONS

By

GEORGE P. SMITH, II

Professor of Law
Catholic University Law School
Washington, D.C.

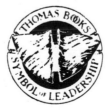

CHARLES C THOMAS • PUBLISHER
Springfield • Illinois • U.S.A.

Published and Distributed Throughout the World by

CHARLES C THOMAS • PUBLISHER
2600 South First Street
Springfield, Illinois 62794-9265

© *1989 by* CHARLES C THOMAS • PUBLISHER

ISBN 0-398-05591-2

Library of Congress Catalog Card Number: 89-4390

With THOMAS BOOKS *careful attention is given to all details of manufacturing
and design. It is the Publisher's desire to present books that are satisfactory as to their
physical qualities and artistic possibilities and appropriate for their particular use.*
THOMAS BOOKS *will be true to those laws of quality that assure a good name
and good will.*

Printed in the United States of America
SC-R-3

Library of Congress Cataloging-in-Publication Data

Smith, George Patrick, 1939–
    Final choices : autonomy in health care decisions / by George P.
Smith II.
      p.   cm.
    Includes bibliographies and index.
    ISBN 0-398-05591-2
    1. Medical ethics.   2. Suicide—Moral and ethical aspects.
3. Euthanasia—Moral and ethical aspects.   4. Right to die—Moral
and ethical aspects.   I. Title.
    [DNLM: 1. Ethics, Medical.   2. Euthanasia.   3. Right to Die.
4. Suicide.   W 50 S648f]
R726.S57   1989
174'.24—dc 19
DNLM/DLC
for Library of Congress   89-4390
                                               CIP

To Martha Biggerstaff Jones
inspirational teacher, valued
friend and surrogate mother.

"I can no other answer make but thanks, and thanks and ever thanks."
William Shakespeare, *TWELFTH NIGHT.*

"... mere living is not a good, but living well. Accordingly, the wise man will live as long as he ought, not as long as he can. He will mark in what place, with whom, and how he is to conduct his existence, and not the quantity, of his life. ... It is not a question of dying earlier or later, but of dying well or ill. And dying well means escape from the danger of living ill." Seneca from EPISTULA MORALES, "On Suicide" in ETHICAL CHOICES at 54 (R. Beck, J. Orr eds. 1970).

"I'm not afraid to die but I am afraid of this illness, what it's doing to me. I'm not better. I'm worse. There's never any relief from it now. Nothing but nausea and this pain. ... Who does it benefit if I die slowly? ... I'm stuck—stuck in life. I don't want to be here anymore. I don't see why I can't get out." B. ROLLIN, LAST WISH 149, 150, 170 (1985).

ACKNOWLEDGMENTS

During my sabbatical in 1984, I began my research and development of this book as a Visiting Fellow at Clare Hall, Cambridge University. To the former President of the Hall, Sir Michael Stoker, I extend my thanks for his good offices that created a conducive atmosphere for contemplation and research. The innumerable kindnesses and friendship of Derek W. Bowett, the Whewell Professor of International Law and former President of Queens' College must also be recognized. I profited from insightful dialogue with Professor Benjy F. Brooks of the University of Texas Health Science Center at Houston, who was in 1984 a Visiting Fellow at Clare Hall, and Andrew Grubb, a Fellow at Fitzwilliam College, Cambridge, concerning my present area of investigation. The resources of the Squire Law Library, the University Library and the Radzinowicz Library of Criminology were made readily accessible thanks in full measure to the efficiency of the Librarian of the Squire, Keith J. A. McVeigh. His indefatigable spirits and high level of professionalism were a joy to behold; and I prospered from both.

When I arrived in Sydney, Australia, to take up my post as Fulbright Visiting Professor of Law and Medical Jurisprudence at the University of New South Wales under an Australian-American Fulbright Foundation Award, my good and valued friend, Dr. George G. Winterton, Chairman of the Law Faculty, had seen to it that everything was in order and ran smoothly during my stay, and for this I thank him most sincerely. The kindness and support of Professor Ivan A. Shearer, the Dean of Law Faculty and to his immediate predecessor, Professor Don Harding, are also acknowledged with pleasure. Four others in Australia must be thanked as well for their consistent encouragement, kind support and friendship: Robert F. Brian, the Law Librarian at the New South Wales Law Faculty; Philip Bates of the Faculty of Health Administration at the University and Russell Scott, the Deputy Chairman of the New South Wales Law Reform Commission and the Honorable Michael D. Kirby, CMG, President, the Court of Appeal, Supreme Court of New South

Wales. Finally, the generous support of the Australian-American Fulbright Foundation is acknowledged sincerely.

During the Summer of 1985, I was a Fellow at the Institute of Advanced Study at Indiana University in Bloomington where I continued my research and began my writing of this book. I thank, most sincerely, Dr. Roger G. Newton, the Director of the Institute, for his assistance and support during an equally pleasant stay. I would again be remiss if I did not acknowledge the encouragement and assistance which I received from Dr. David H. Smith and the Poynter Center for the Study of Ethics and American Institutions, of which he is the Director, during my very enjoyable Summer in Bloomington.

In December, 1986, and again in May, 1987, I was a Visiting Fellow at the American Bar Foundation in Chicago. To William L. F. Felstiner, Esquire, the Executive Director of the Foundation, I extend my large debt of gratitude for his assistance and support. The facilities of the Foundation were indispensable to me at a most critical juncture in my preparation of this book.

In July, 1988, I was a Visiting Fellow at the McGill University Centre for Medicine, Ethics and Law in Montreal and there finalized my work on this book. To Professor Margaret A. Sommerville, the Director of the Centre, I extend my sincere thanks for her support and friendship.

INTRODUCTION

It is estimated that someone in the United States commits suicide every nineteen minutes.[1] Yet, owing to the fact that it is often quite difficult to distinguish suicide from an accidental or natural death (particularly among the elderly), precise data is scarce.[2] Indeed, most experts are of the opinion that suicide is underreported.[3] This is the case primarily because attending physicians and involved families often tend to co-operate in disguising or ignoring the less than obvious suicides—particularly so with older persons in order to avoid various social stigmas being attached to the surviving relatives.[4]

Suicide may be defined "as doing something which results in one's death, either from the intention of ending one's life or the intention to bring about some other state of affairs (such as relief from pain) which one thinks it certain or highly probably can be achieved only by means of death or will produce death.[5] Since death is a necessary element of suicide, reflexive descriptions of death are important to allow a full understanding of the very term, suicide. Thus one description would be simply that one has killed himself; another would be that one has let himself be killed. Additionally, one might choose a suicide by deliberately—with premediation—taking his own life, or by ordering an agent to accomplish the act and thereby *getting himself killed.* By falling into a pool and refusing to swim in order to save himself, an individual could *let himself be killed.* He could even kill himself by providing a physical confrontation, proceeding to offer little resistance and defense and thereby letting himself be killed (as intended). For a suicide to occur, then, the deceased must kill himself, get killed or let himself be killed.[6] As can be seen, suicide as a form of behavior has developed its own particular praxis.

Voluntary euthanasia has been variously described as "assisted suicide,"[7] and "within the knife's edge between suicide and murder."[8] Suicide can be even self-administered euthanasia.[9] Thus, the principal conundrum resulting here is determining if an act of euthanasia is voluntary whether in turn it should be regarded as a suicide or as a murder? And the morality of euthanasia becomes inextricably linked to that of suicide. More specifically, if committing suicide were no longer regarded as a tendentious expression and the very act, itself, were recognized as but an exercise of enlightened self-determination, so too would euthanasia be similarly re-classified. These simple changes in the taxonomy of these two words would, in turn, hopefully give rise to a new attitude toward both life and death. Instead of cheapening life[10] and viewing it as but a casual or inconsequential occurrence, this re-thinking would show a new sensitivity to the quality of life. It would not promote a passionate desire for death but for independence, honesty and integrity. Human disposal would not be the end sought here. Rather, the goal would be "the enhancement of human dignity by permitting each man's last act to be an exercise of his free choice between a tortured, hideous death and a painless dignified one."[11]

Dating from at least the seventeenth century, rational suicide has been recognized as a concept or phenomenon.[12] It has been suggested that the rationality of a suicidal act would tie to the very rationality of the philosophy recognized as guiding the deliberations of individuals contemplating the act.[13] Defining rationality as a logical means of problem solving which have proven to be reliable over the course of time, the rationality of one's philosophy is tested not only by the degree to which it is free of mysticism but by the degree of self-criticism it has undergone by the decision maker.[14] Accordingly, should the philosophy in question embody a set of institutionalized political or religious beliefs, the decision maker must evaluate critically the very institutions wherein these beliefs are set if rational judgment is to be acquired.[15] While this principle is clear, its practice and application are extremely difficult to realize.[16] Within the context of suicide, "a rational decision is the one in favor of the life course which one would prefer, comparing death with the best option open to one if he had the alternatives correctly and vividly before him in a normal frame of mind."[17]

Contrariwise, irrational suicide would give rise or be exampled in a case where an individual in a state of despair abandons totally any serious commitment to make rational decisions on the basis of future consequences of subsequent actions.[18] Oftentimes, human commitments may require a kind of irrationality if they are in fact to be respected (e.g., unfathomable grief or mourning over the loss of a spouse; unrequited "first" loves of teenagers).[19]

Suicide, as a concept, is—as death—forever changing.[20] Although the "badness" of death is debatable,[21] most members of today's society would hold that suicide is—indeed—bad or improper,[22] and that so too is euthanasia.[23] Life is not as an amaranth or imaginary flower that never fades. For all too many, with the "benefits" of modern medicine and treatment, the fading process is extended with tragic withering, discoloration and odor. The current controversy surrounding the right to refuse treatment for a terminally or non-terminal competent or incompetent individual has both its genesis and its nexus in the central objection to an individual's exercise of his right of self-determination through suicide or euthanasia. Refusing necessary life sustaining treatment has been declared to be a "form of suicide,"[24] and its recognition and allowance as "modern paganism."[25]

In order to clarify the issues and dispel the inherent confusion over this point of contention and thereby postulate a construct to facilitate contemporary health care decision making, I have advocated a seemingly simple—but admittedly complex—change in both the attitude and the very definition of suicide and euthanasia. The forces at work to effect this change are to be found in the courts and state legislative bodies as well as in professional organizations such as the American Medical Association and the former President's Commission for The Study of Ethical Problems in Medicine and Biomedical and Behavioral Research. They will be explored and critically analyzed in order to determine whether they are responsive to the growing societal demands or but recalcitrant and unreasonable initiatives and without reason or popular support.

These mechanisms will be seen as providing a framework for principled decision making that is grounded in actions designed to recognize humaness, love and compassion, the best interest of the at-risk patient or competent individual and the state interest in preserving life, and the costs and benefits of the action in question and thus its reasonableness.[26] They in turn will all conduce to a basic recognition and application of an enlightened self-determination. Questions of ethical, moral and philosophical and religious consistency are inextricably related to any legal analysis of the issue and are recognized and analyzed as dynamic vectors of force in the entire decision making process. Their influence oftentimes will be seen as more confusing than as unifying.

Whether a right to decline life sustaining treatment implies an equal liberty or co-ordinate right to commit suicide and effect euthanasia should not be regarded as an issue of crucial concern; for it is not necessary to attempt to draw a hard and fast line between suicide and a refusal of treatment decision. The major point to be made and the central recognition sought is that competent persons within either of these contexts should have both a moral and legal right—acting for whatever purposes—to refuse life-sustaining medical treatment.[27] And, furthermore, as part of a *treatment* refusal, total parenteral nutrition, feeding gastrostomies, nasogastric tubes and all other means of providing alimentation should not be required.[28]

Since generally most of the states have decriminalized suicide and seldom enforce prohibitions against assisting it,[29] under my new proposal for an unfettered recognition of a right to enlightened self-determination, this shallow statutory ruse would be abolished.[30] Perhaps the issue of rational suicide is more tolerable or understandable if it is but viewed as a limiting case of the right to be left alone and to choose the circumstances under which treatment will be followed.[31]

In line with my primary proposal for reclassification of terms, is one designed to similarly re-cast euthanasia so that it too is definitionally and attitudinally consistent with the new principle of self-determination and thus decriminalized. What is regarded as passive euthanasia is already practiced widely and seldom prosecuted.[32] If voluntary active euthanasia were not de-criminalized as a consequence of the re-classification scheme propounded, then surely an immunity from prosecution should be allowed for those assisting in allowing a competent or incompetent individual to complete such an act of self-determination. Alternatively, the traditional concept of euthanasia could be allowed as an affirmative defense to a charge of murder and accepted if the participating parties acted in good faith.[33]

The central purpose of this book is to show that by allowing one's determination of his own life plan and thus his pursuit of the good of that plan, not only is full substance to the concept of liberty acknowledged[34] but a further recognition and advancement of the understanding that the very endowment of free will is "the basis of our right to individual freedom of action, the right to carry into execution the things we freely choose to do" achieved.[35]

ENDNOTES

1. Mansfield, Focus: Suicide, Wash. Post, Dec. 3, 1982, at E5, col. 3.

In order to express the national concern over the growing problem of suicide, on October 7, 1987, House Concurrent Resolution 194 was introduced expressing, as such, "the sense of the Congress that efforts to allow people to assist others to commit suicide and efforts to promote suicide as a rational solution to certain problems should be opposed."

2. Colburn, Death by Choice: Nathan Pritikin's Suicide and The Critical Problem Affecting Aging Men, Health Mag., Wash. Post, Feb. 27, 1985 at 7.

3. Id.

4. Id.

5. Brandt, The Rationality of Suicide in SUICIDE: THE PHILOSOPHICAL ISSUES at 117, 118 (M. BATTIN, D. MAYO eds. 1980).

6. Windt, The Concept of Suicide in SUICIDE: THE PHILOSOPHICAL ISSUES 39 at 41 (M. BATTIN, D. MAYO eds. 1980).

7. Gillon, Suicide and Voluntary Euthanasia: Historical Perspective in EUTHANASIA AND THE RIGHT TO DIE at 181 (A. Downing ed. 1969).

8. McClanahan, The Patient's Right to Die: Moral and Spiritual Aspects of Euthanasia, 38 MEMPHIS MED. J. 303 (1963).

9. See G. Grisez, J. M. Boyle, Jr., LIFE AND DEATH WITH LIBERTY AND JUSTICE, Ch. 5 (1979).

Refusing necessary treatment is a form of suicide just as a hunger strike. Yet, "the only form of suicide to which the law can attach a penalty for the attempt is suicide by an affirmative act." C. RICE, THE VANISHING RIGHT TO LIVE 83 (1969).

10. Rise, supra at 79.

11. Giancola, The Discontinuance of Extraordinary Medical Treatment from a Terminal Patient, 1980 MED. TRIAL TECH. Q. 326, 342.

12. Motto, The Right to Suicide: A Psychiatrists View in SUICIDE: The Philosophical Issues 212 at 215 (M. Battin, D. Mayo eds. 1980).

13. Id.

It has been stated that logical suicide is often but the simple expression of philosophical pessimism. J. MEERLOO, SUICIDE AND MASS SUICIDE 111 (1962).

14. Id.

15. Id.

16. Id.

17. Brandt, The Morality and Rationality of Suicide in SUCIODOLOGY: CONTEMPORARY DEVELOPMENTS Ch. 12 at 391 (E. Sheidman ed. 1976).

Judgments about the rationality of suicide depend upon an assessment of alternative states of affairs and their probability (e.g., painful progression of a terminal illness). J. CHILDRESS, WHO SHOULD DECIDE? PATERNALISM IN HEALTH CARE 159 (1982).

Public television presented a case documentary in June, 1980, on Jo Roman—a

New York City artist and writer—who undertook, with family support, rational suicide in order to avoid protracted suffering from cancer. "Rational Suicide" Raises Patient Rights Issues, 66 A.B.A.J. 1499 (1980); TIME Mag., July 7, 1980, at 49.

18. Mayo, Irrational Suicide in SUICIDE: THE PHILOSOPHICAL ISSUES at 133–135 (M. Battin, D. Mayo eds. 1980).

See also, Brandt, The Rationality of Suicide in SUICIDE: THE PHILO-SOPHICAL ISSUES at 127 (M. Battin, D. Mayo eds. 1980).

19. Id.

20. J. MEERLOO, SUICIDE AND MASS SUICIDE 111 (1962).

21. See T. NAGEL, MORAL QUESTIONS 1 (1976).

22. See generally, SUICIDE: THE PHILOSOPHICAL ISSUES (M. BATTIN, D. MAYO eds. 1980).

23. See generally Kuhse, The Case for Voluntary Euthanasia, 14 LAW, MED. & HEALTH CARE 145 (1986).

24. C. RICE, THE VANISHING RIGHT TO LIVE 83 (1969).

25. Brophy v. New England Siani Hosp., Inc., 398 Mass. 417, 497 N.E. 2d 626 at 640 (1986), Nolan, J. dissenting.

26. See G. SMITH, GENETICS, ETHICS AND THE LAW 2, 8, 164 (1981).

27. J. CHILDRESS, WHO SHOULD DECIDE? PATERNALISM IN HEALTH CARE 163 (1982).

28. See Paris & McCormick, The Catholic Tradition on The Use of Nutrients and Fluids, AMERICA 2 (May 2, 1987).

29. See Engelhardt & Malloy, Suicide and Assisting Suicide: A Critique of Legal Sanctions, 36 S. W. L. J. 1003, 1019, 1120 (1982); Survey, Euthanasia: Criminal, Tort, Constitutional and Legislative Considerations, 48 NOTRE DAME L. REV. 1202, 1206 (1973).

30. See M. HEIFETZ, THE RIGHT TO DIE 97–98 (1975) for analysis of another construct for validating suicide.

31. Engelhardt, Suicide and The Cancer Patient, 36 CA–A CANCER J. FOR CLINICIANS 105 (Mar.–Apr. 1986).

32. Rational Suicide Raises Rights Issue, 66 A.B.A.J. 1499, 1501 (1980).

See also, G. GRISEZ, J. BOYLE, JR., LIFE AND DEATH WITH LIBERTY AND JUSTICE 136–138 (1979).

33. See G. WILLIAMS, THE SANCTITY OF LIFE AND THE CRIMINAL LAW, Ch. at 340 (1958).

34. C. FRIED, RIGHT AND WRONG 146–147 (1978).

35. M. ADLER, WE HOLD THESE TRUTHS 123 (1987).

CONTENTS

FINAL CHOICES
AUTONOMY IN
HEALTH CARE DECISIONS

Chapter I

THE ETIOLOGY OF SUICIDE

PSYCHOLOGICAL AND HISTORICAL UNDERPINNINGS

While there are one hundred and forty possible causes of death, only four modes have been recognized: natural, accident, suicide and homicide.[1] It has been suggested that a more meaningful and accurate classification would be to consider the role of the individual in his own act of self-destruction as being: intentional, subintentional (or those cases where an individual plays a partial or unconscious role in promoting his own death) or unintentional.[2]

Suicide, as a word, is thought to have originated either in Sir Thomas Browne's RELIGIO MEDICI written in 1635 or in 1651 by Walter Charleton.[3] "Suicidology" was used independently in the 1960's as a word to explain, scientifically, the study of the phenomena of suicide.[4] The term, "suicide," is applied to all those cases of death that result directly or indirectly from either a positive or a negative act of the victim himself — which he in turn knows or has reason to know will produce this desired result.[5]

Though one may be reconciled to the prospect of his own death, this does not — in turn — mean that he is in fact reconciled to death itself as one of those inescapable facts of the human condition.[6] Depending upon the mores and the traditions of each society, from an historical standpoint suicide has been not only acclaimed and despised, but sought after and feared.[7]

It has been postulated that suicide is to be viewed properly as an attenuated homicide and provides a great advantage to society because it allows for a way of ridding it of numbers "of useless or harmful persons without social intervention" and in a simple and economical manner.[8] The telling question, then, is put in this form: "Is it not better to let them put themselves out of the way voluntarily and quietly, than to force society to eject them from its midst by violence?"[9]

Durkheim found the aetiology of suicide in: "abnormal psychology;

social psychology; anthropology; meteorological and other cosmic factors; religion; marriage; the family; divorce; primitive rites and customs; social and economic crimes; crime, law and jurisprudence and in history, education, and occupational groups."[10] In a very real sense, then, suicide is a social phenomenon.[11]

As suicide has come to be viewed, over time, as symptomatic of individual psychopathology together with social disorganization, its philosophical underpinnings were neglected for legal and scientific analysis.[12] Today, scholars are now recognizing the inextricable relationship that exists among law, philosophy and medical science as vectors of dynamic force in both the theory and application of suicide.[13] This recognition is, in large part, owing to the fact of the rapid development of new sophisticated medical technologies that allow the extension of human life beyond the limits desired by the at-risk individual and his affected family and the acceptance of voluntary euthanasia, itself a form of suicide, as a valid alternative to intolerable pain, suffering and economic depletion.[14]

The hard questions of suicide are, in reality, the hard questions of death control and management; for any analysis of the morality, the rationality and the very right of self-determination to die are tied inextricably to a plethora of complex medical and non-medical areas such as the competent and the incompetent individual's refusal of lifesaving medical treatment, informed consent to potentially lethal experimental studies and fatal organ donations, as well as destructive behavior such as alcohol and cigarette smoking.[15] Inevitably, autonomy and self-determination become watchwords for death with dignity.

There is no clear passage within the Old Testament propounding an explicit view of the ancient Judaic view on suicide,[16] with only eight cases of acts that might properly be considered suicide being reported.[17] As in the New Testament, the Old Testament does not contain any explicit prohibition against suicide.[18] Although cultural prohibitions against suicide may have acted as a restraint on suicides with the Hebrews, it has been suggested that the infrequency of suicides was more correctly viewed as due to the centrality of positivism within the religious tenets of the faith that placed not only a high value on life itself but acknowledged a special providential commitment of God to them as a people.[19]

Neither the Greek nor Roman laws were concerned uniquely with suicide—except when the act was one of a slave or of a soldier.[20] The penalties for such acts were the forfeiture of all personality owned previously by the suicidee and the confiscation of his estates—thereby preventing their passage to the heirs of the estate.[21] For Greco-Roman physicians, assisted suicides were a common place activity and regarded as acts outside the scope and the interest of the law.[22] Indeed, for the Platonists, Cynics and Stoics, the act of suicide was considered "an honorable alternative to hopeless illness."[23]

Open toleration of suicide may be viewed as commencing with the Greek culture.[24] The toleration was for the act when it was undertaken for nobility of purpose:[25] as an expression of grief, high patriotic principle or to avoid dishonor.[26] Moderation and high principle were the keys to this acceptant view; wantonness was not condoned.[27] The "acceptance" of suicide as a rational act came with the Romans, particularly through Greek Stoic philosophy, which made suicide into the most reasonable and desirable of all ways to end life.[28] Both the Stoics and the Epicureans claimed to be as indifferent to death as to life.[29] For the Epicureans, the principle was pleasure; whatever promoted that was good and whatever produced pain was evil.[30] For the Stoics, the ideal was more vague, more dignified: that of life in accordance with nature.[31] When it no longer seemed to be so, then death came as a rational choice befitting a rational nature.[32]

The Greek Stoics had developed a rational attitude toward suicide that conformed to their ideal of life in accordance with nature. The advanced Stoicism of the later Roman Empire internalized these beliefs.[33] Now the dilemma to be faced was when the inner compulsion became intolerable, the question was no longer whether or not one should kill himself, but how to do so with the greatest dignity, bravery and style.[34] Stated otherwise, it was an achievement of the Greeks to divest suicide of all primitive horrors and then gradually to discuss the subject more or less rationally, in an objective unemotional manner.[35] The Romans, however, reinvested it with emotion—but in doing so, turned the emotions upside down.[36] Thus, suicide was no longer morally evil; to the contrary, one's manner of going became but a practical test of excellence and of virtue.[37] Indeed, the manner in which a Roman died was viewed as the measure of ultimate value of life.[38]

The early Christians also showed an indifference to death—but from a different perspective.[39] Since life, itself, was unimportant—in that the world only tempted one to sin—death was a welcome blessing. Stated otherwise, the more the Church expressed its view that the world was full of sin and temptation and man waits only on earth until his death releases him to heavenly glory, the more irresistable the temptation to suicide became.[40]

Because of a growing confusion regarding discernable distinctions between approved and glorified martyrdom and ignominious acts of suicide, St. Augustine, who lived from 354–430 A.D., spoke out in condemnation of suicide even when such acts were being condoned by the Stoics for those Christian women who had been violated by invading barbarians.[41] Augustine considered suicide, or self-imposed death, from a number of perspectives and concluded that the act was sinful because of its violation of the Sixth Commandment: namely, "Thou shall not kill."[42] He did admit of two circumstances where self-imposed death would be tolerated: specifically when performed validly by the state — as in war and as an exercise of capital punishment and by special intimation by God — as with the death of certain individuals such as Abraham and Samson.[43] No authority reposed within the individual to take his own life, however.[44]

In the Middle Ages, it was for St. Thomas Aquinas who, as did St. Augustine, to proclaim that self-imposed death, or suicide, is always to be regarded as sinful.[45] With the Renaissance and the Reformation and the turn of the century, unyielding opposition to suicide began to errode — sparked primarily by the publication of THE ANATOMY OF MELAN-CHOLY in 1621 by Robert Burton and BIATHANTOS in 1646 by John Donne.[46]

Both the opponents and the defenders of suicide found themselves in the eighteenth century still adrift philosophically with no one, distinct position regarding the issue in evidence.[47] It remained for David Hume and Immanuel Kant to polarize thought by their analyses of this issue. It is far beyond the scope of this book and this brief historical overview to probe the underpinnings of the philosophies of these two men. Suffice it to state, succinctly, that, as an empiricist, Hume determined the foundation of morality was to be found in a "natural sentiment that distinguishes the good and the bad."[48] This foundation could not be based on God, because verification of his existence was lacking.[49] If an obligation undertaken involved the promotion or endurance of great suffering, society could not be properly understood as being entitled to extract it from the individual, himself.[50] Accordingly, if one's life promoted no type of mutual benefit for either the individual or society, and so-called moral imperative to continue that life would fail.[51]

For Kant, the foundation of morality was tied to the nature of the human person.[52] Although he espoused self-sacrifice, observing that it was better "to sacrifice one's life rather than one's morality," he would not have this idea confused with suicide.[53] Committing suicide was, for Kant, an immoral act because,

> If he destroys himself in order to escape from painful circumstances, he uses a person merely as a means to maintain a tolerable condition up to the end of life. But a man is not a thing.... To destroy the subject of morality in his own person is tantamount to obliterating from the world, as far as he can, the very existence of morality itself.[54]

In 1854, the common law courts of England first recognized the criminality of suicide.[55] Although no clear answer is provided that accounts for the delay for this action—since it would follow that if suicide were a crime acts of attempted suicide would also be punishable—it has been posited that instead of structuring a deliberate penal policy against such acts, the courts responded to a mechanism utilized by the medieval judges to enrich the coffers of the treasury.[56]

In the mid 1700's in England, the punishment for suicide was forfeiture and confiscation of the suicides personal property by the Crown, although all real property was allowed to pass to the heirs of the decedent's estate.[57] In 1870, however, with the enactment of the Forfeiture Act, forefeitures for suicides were abolished.[58] With the Suicide Act of 1961,[59] acts of suicide and attempted suicides were de-criminalized—although complicity in another's suicide remains a felony.[60]

From the colonial period in America through the 1970's, a clear demonstration is seen of society's dominant attitude against suicide.[61] Whether the American colonies adopted *in toto* the Common Law of England regarding the criminalization of suicide when they were formed is open to historical debate.[62] What can be stated, however, is that by the 19th century suicide, in America, was not regarded—in a practical sense—a criminal offense.[63] Today, a majority of the states—twenty-six together with the Commonwealth of Puerto Rico—have statutes that prohibit assisting suicide.[64] Three other states appear to hold an individual who assists a suicide as a principal to murder.[65] Relying upon the common laws of crimes,[66] it is thought that Maryland[67] and Massachusetts[68] would also penalize assisting suicide. It is less certain whether Alabama,[69] the District of Columbia,[70] West Virginia,[71] Virginia[72] and Tennessee,[73] would follow suit. While Hawaii[74] and Indiana[75] treat acts of causing suicide as punishable offenses, they do not prohibit the act of assisting it. Nine other states have no such prohibitions.[76] Yet, prosecutions for either aiding or abetting suicide are quite rare.[77]

In summary, then, it can be seen that in a number of American jurisdictions neither acts of suicide nor assistance thereto have been punished. Yet, in others, attempted suicide has been criminalized. Interestingly, the majority of jurisdictions in the United States have—since the Nation's founding—imposed no criminal sanction upon those successful or unsuccessful undertakings by individuals who wish to end their lives.[78]

Attitudinal Variances About Death

Philippe Aries, the noted French social historian, has identified and charted three phases in the development of Western attitudes toward death.[79] Death was seen, in the Middle Ages, as an unexceptional and—indeed—impersonal event, yet neutralized by the Christian belief in immortality and accepted by the community at large with a simple resignation.[80] The phrase, *"et moriemur"*—and we shall die—characterized this attitude. A dramatic change occurred around the twentieth century with the recognition of the individual's importance—for with this came a much more personal conception of death. Thus, man insisted upon participating in his own death because, quite simply, he saw it as a truly exceptional moment in time; the moment that gave his own individuality a definite, observable form.[81] The logic offered here was that if one were to be master of his own life, then obviously he must be master of his own death, *"la mort de soi."* Curiously, in the traditional death bed scene of this period, the dying person became the principal character presiding over the proceedings—yet the event was treated by onlookers in a matter-of-fact manner. Accordingly, mourning tended to be quite conventional and, by standards of the later centuries, perfunctory.[82]

The seventeenth century gave rise to the possibility of one sharing his death with his family and friends—with all concerned parties participating in the decision making process of the dying person; whereas in the past these matters were solely of the concern of the afflicted person, himself.[83] Interestingly, by the middle of the eighteenth century, a new attitude concerning death had arisen: *"la mort de ton"*—or thy death. Thus, the onlookers in a death-bed scene now assumed a greater responsibility and were expected, to a much greater extent than heretofore, to observe *and* act upon the dying person's wishes and—most importantly—to preserve his memory.[84] The hope of living forever in the memory of posterity, took form in the architecture and iconography of tombs as the medium of remembrance—with cemeteries more or less becoming museums.[85]

Toynbee suggests that attitudes toward death have been changing, in the modern western world, over the last three hundred years as a consequence of the "contemporary progressive recession . . . of the beliefs in the tenets of Christianity."[86] An honest belief in Christian doctrine—that includes a belief in the personal immortality of human souls—is obviously something more than a mere intellectual acknowledgement of a set of theological propositions; for it involves an *auto de fe* which thereby commits the believer to action not only on a moral and spiritual plane, but on an intellectual one as well. In a word, "It commits him . . . to the Christian attitude towards death.[87]

In the West, and particularly so in the United States, the word, "death," has until rather recently within the last twenty years or so, been regarded as almost an unmentionable word.[88] Indeed, the quest for immortality has gained new momentum with the efforts of some to defy death by utilizing a deep-freeze process known as cryonic suspension designed as such to suspend the bodily processes at "death" until resuscitation can be undertaken at a later time.[89] For all these shifts in attitudes, death is still regarded as "un-American," with preferences being given to less demanding word usages such as "pass on" or "pass away" than to "die" or "death."[90] And, tragically, there is still a marked reluctance to advise a dying person that he is dying.[91] The exaggerated and almost simpleminded insistence on physical continuance and the maintenance thereof with all means necessary—regardless of the qualitative condition in which life is pursued is childish and narcissistic. Such an obsession distracts "the soul's natural quest. It is a distraction from the duty to master the fine art of living well, which requires rising above concern for mere bodily continuance."[92] Acceptance of death should be viewed "as an inherent to life and happiness" and "belongs to normal life."[93]

CONTEMPORARY CAUSES AND CONCERNS

Suicide has become a common fact of life. Many explanations have been offered to present an understanding of it. One such position was, in 1840, that the increasing numbers of suicide of that day were due in large part to socialism.[94] And, to fortify this point, the fact that, upon the publication of Tom Paine's, AGE OF REASON, sudden increases in suicides were recorded was submitted as evidence of the major conclusion.[95] Other causative factors including "atmospherical moisture" and "masturbation" were listed as well.[96] Indeed, masturbation was to be viewed as "a certain secret vice which, we are afraid, is practiced to an enormous extent in our public schools."[97] Two major cures designed to stem suicidal urges were cold showers and laxatives.[98] Another popular belief was that suicide was an act undertaken largely by young lovers.[99] Others sought to explain it away by viewing it as a "national habit" which descended upon some people as a plague might.[100] President Dwight Eisenhower even went too far as to express his belief that the high suicide rate in Sweden was an uncontroverted example of the ravages of uncontrolled social welfare.[101]

Perhaps the most common denominator of suicides is loneliness, a motive arising from marital discord, sickness, unrequited love affairs, and from social factors such as unemployment, divorce, widowhood and imprisonment.[102] Loneliness and interpersonal conflicts are properly considered as motives for suicides—not causes. Rather, the causes of suicide are to be reckoned as "the biophysical driving forces, which often do not even rise to the consciousness of the individual and thus cannot constitute motives, but which are related to race, age, sex, work and social status."[103] Whatever may, within the taxonomy of suicide behavior, be classified as motives and causes, what is known for a fact is that those who seek to complete the act, itself, often complain that either their lives no longer have meaning or they are no longer "worth living."[104] They no longer have a sense of self-mastery in their lives because of failures in interpersonal relations and economic pursuits and an inability to thus redefine situational arrangements.[105]

Another explanation proferred here is that one can inherit certain hereditary vulnerabilities toward suicide.[106] Sociobiologists and behavioral ecologists in fact stress the biological perspective—and specifically human biological adaption—as the determinative factor in understanding and dealing with the issues of suicide. Accordingly, this perspective simply subsumes the other theories or disciplines advanced by sociology, psychodynamic models, anthropology, cognition and learning and physiology under it as an explanatory process.[107]

While it may be difficult to discover a common denominator that can explain suicide as resulting from a conscious rational process,[108] Durkheim has implied that when an option for suicide is made, the individual responding thusly has made a "conscious-rational choice" drawn from and built upon a basis of motives actually founded in reality."[109] And, interestingly, the vast majority of all members of society has—at one time or other—"played" with the idea of committing suicide.[110] This fact is indeed consistent with Freud's *Destrudo* or death drive which he found in man.[111] "Man's inner destructibility is, like every instinctual tendency, rooted in both the primary drive to live and in its opposite—the tendency to return to the inorganic matrix."[112]

In a majority of suicides studied in the United States, the two most common disorders found afflicting most Americans were depression and chronic alcoholism.[113] Owing to the fact that oftentimes a physician—during an office visit or telephone consultation with a patient—neglects to prove to either the patient or his family more fully about a present medical problem and depression and alcoholism go undiagnosed. Yet, oftentimes, they are diagnosed but not treated vigorously by either actual hospitalization, drug therapy or, when that fails, electroconvulsive therapy.[114] It can be hoped that with improved methods of treatment, heightened recognition of the symptomology or etiology of suicide and the growth of suicide-prevention and crisis-intervention services will eventually curtail the incidence of suicide.[115]

Since most Americans choosing suicide elect to complete the act by use of a firearm (and more specifically handguns), it could be argued—finally, that restricting the use of handgun availability would have the end result of allowing fewer Americans to commit suicide.[116] Interestingly, in those states where there are strict gun control laws, a lower suicide rate is recorded.[117]

The Elderly

The elderly who commit suicide are not dramatically different in type from the younger teenagers in that loss of health or reverses in economic affairs promotes an inescapable sense of hopelessness.[118] The principal difference between the age groups is that the elderly succeed in their mission more often than others, with studies indicating a ratio of attempts to completions among fifteen to twenty-four year olds as high as 200 to 1 while in the over sixty-five year old age groups, the ratio is four to one.[119]

For the older and socially isolated, the intent to die is more genuine and the choice of methods to effect that end is more lethal.[120] Normally, three scenarios have been found to be common with dual suicides or murder-suicides.[121] The first proffers the explanation: "You're dying, and I love you too much to exist without you."[122] In the second, a gravely ill wife who knows that she is dying asks her husband to kill her, as she is unable to carry out the act itself. If the husband acquiesces, he could face a murder sentence or extended imprisonment and, thus, may take his own life as well.[123] The third scenario is one of inadvertence because one of the spouses did not intend to die.[124] Accordingly, a distressed or physically ill husband, for example, may murder his wife with the purpose of actually sparing her from either losing him or being abandoned after he has departed. In effect, what he is saying is: "Life will be much worse for you when I die, so I'm going to spare you from that pain by killing you now. After I've done that, I can kill myself."[125]

It has been suggested that a central element in reducing the continuing use of these scenarios is to be found by re-doubling efforts to assure the elderly of a still meaningful societal role once they have retired and assure them that once one spouse dies, the other will not be discounted or disgarded.[126] Whether the heavy commitment in economic support needed to make these assurances is questionable at best. Indeed, at this point in time, health care expenses for the elderly are so astronomical that unless the average retired elderly couple has had the foresight to make solid financial plans for their future, upon the death of one spouse, the surviving spouse may indeed find herself largely discounted or discarded.

Teenagers

Of particular disturbance is the rather dramatic problem seen in teenage suicides. Whether a real or fabricated crisis exists is debatable.[127] Although the 1960's and early 1970's saw a dramatic increase in the actual number of suicides committed by youths, even in 1975—considered as the peak year for teenage suicides—the total number of ten to fourteen year olds committing suicide was 11,594.[128]

> Viewed internationally, the American problem is not a crisis. Among young males, the U.S. suicide rates of 19.7 per 100,000 teenagers is below the rates found in Switzerland (33.5), West Germany (21.2) and Norway (20.2). For young women, the American rate (4.6) also falls below that found in Denmark (5.0) France (5.0) and Japan (6.4).[129]

Even though these statistics and the assurance that they are, at least to the United States, not of crisis dimension, it is of concern to learn—for example—that thirty-one percent of high achieving teenagers listed in WHO'S WHO AMONG AMERICAN HIGH SCHOOL STUDENTS (drawn from a population survey of 1,943 such students) have actually contemplated suicide and four percent have in fact attempted it.[130] The same survey also discovered that seventy-one percent of those surveyed suggested that suicides for this particular age group could be prevented effectively not only through so-called suicide awareness programs for teenagers and parents, but by counseling in schools, more direct involvement between parents and teacher-counselors, and crisis-prevention hot lines—to name but several of the most important.[131] Of those surveyed, the factors listed as most contributive to suicide were:

> Feelings of personal worthlessness, 86 percent; feelings of isolation and loneliness, 81 percent; pressure to achieve, 72 percent; fear of failure, 61 percent; drug and alcohol use, 58 percent; communication with parents, 58 percent; actual failure, 56 percent; lack of attention from parents, 50 percent; lack of stability in the family, 49 percent; fear for personal future, 41 percent; unwanted pregnancy, 32 percent; parental divorce, 24 percent; sexual problems, 23 percent; financial concerns, 14 percent.[132]

When four Bergenfield, New Jersey, youths successfully committed a pact suicide on March 11, 1986, wide national news coverage of this event "seems to have had a strong impact on other teenagers," for there were some thirty-five similarly related cases during the succeeding four weeks.[133] Research undertaken at the University of California at San Diego of more than 12,500 teen-age suicides between 1973 and 1979 found that " 'the national rate of suicide among teen-agers rises significantly just after television news or feature stories about suicide,' with the increase proportional to the amount of network coverage."[134] A similarly focused study restricted to the greater New York City area and undertaken by a research team from Columbia University found that in two week periods following the airing of three of four television fictional movies on the subject of suicide, both in the Fall and the Winter of 1984, 1985, respectively, found both suicide attempts and actual completions increased.[135]

Suicide "contagions" and "clusters" can be abated—it is suggested by some—by presenting news stories about suicides in a negative, even gruesome, manner instead of in a neutral or sympathetic posture.[136] Since research suggests front-page stories have a more significant impact on its readers than those on the inside pages.[137] Coverage of suicides should be written in such a manner as to suggest that the suicidees could have, of course, either spoken to a counselor, friend, priest or rabbi or called a listed suicide prevention hot line in order to receive counseling over the issue that precipitated the tragic incident.[138]

If a teenager is of the opinion that death would be beneficial, should he be recognized as having a right to end his life with assistance or autonomously? It has been suggested that for teenagers with either catastrophic illnesses or severe mental impairments, this right of self-determination should be preserved.[139] Obviously, if such recognition of a right — qualified or otherwise, or a policy — were to be held as applicable to unemancipated teenagers who had not reached majority, it would have to be fashioned along the lines as would be done for an incompetent; that is, either a family member (e.g., father, mother, brother, sister or grandparent) or — if none exist — a close personal friend would have to be allowed to have the legal responsibility to determine, acting in concert with the attending physician, whether actions of enlightened self-determination — thereby consistent with the person in question's best interests — were to be undertaken. For the emancipated teenager, his status would be akin to that of any other competent individual of majority and, thus, consistent with present law, be allowed to refuse treatment. The mechanisms for promoting or, as the case may be, implementing this policy of enlightened self-determination will be developed in chapters four and five of this book.

INDIRECT SELF-DESTRUCTIVE BEHAVIORS

Indirect self-destructive behavior comes in many forms: hyper-obesity, smoking, drug and alcohol addiction (substance abuse), motorcycle and auto racing and skydiving — to list but a few.[140] This type of overt behavior distinguishes itself from direct self-destruction by two specific criteria: time and awareness. Thus, since the effect of this indirect behavior is long range and spans a period of years, the person exhibiting the behavior pattern is either unaware of the effects of his actions or simply does not care. But in no case does he consider himself a suicide nor does society seek to commit him involuntarily for restraint of these actions.[141]

The concept of indirect self-destructive behavior, then, is so broad that it embraces not only self-punishment for minor risks merging on a continuum of escalating danger with more serious injuries and — ultimately — death as the outcome.[142] Yet, its essential function is to "deny helplessness and replace it with coping mechanisms that in theory enhance self-esteem."[143] Accordingly, cigarette smoking may allow one to have a feeling of security reinforced yet still permit "one to spit smoke in the face of the world."[144] It has been suggested that all individuals—to one degree or other—seek to deny their utter helplessness against bad luck, fate, death and inner turmoil and indulge in some form of indirect self-destructive behavior which of course society must absorb the costs connected therewith.[145]

Generally, indirect self-destruction proceeds so slowly that it is often taken to be unctuous. Therefore, an individual may damage himself by overeating, seeking stress, neglecting physical fitness, drinking alcohol excessively, or choosing to forego treatment when an illness is contracted.[146] Alcoholism and drug addiction have, in fact, been characterized simply as forms of "slow suicide."[147]

Seeking the pursuit of pleasure, many young males have been found to engage themselves, during their leisure, in high-risk sports which yield high mortality figures. Although reliable statistics are difficult to obtain that document both the frequency of injuries and fatalities for the fifteen to forty year old age group, The Metropolitan Life Insurance Company has presented some interesting statistics for the United States.[148] In 1976, of the almost 400,000 motor vehicle racing drivers on record, 145,000 were drag racers, 115,000 motorcycle racers and 28,000 stock car racers. From 1967 to 1976, inclusive, 436 fatalities from motor vehicle racing were recorded—which included 104 from stock car racing, 77 from motorcycle racing and 74 from automobile drag racing. Interestingly, in 1975, approximately 700 balloon pilots were registered, and from 1964 through 1974, only 16 fatalities resulted from balloon flying. Thirty thousand people had delta kites or hang gliders by 1975 and eighty-five fatalities had resulted from these flights. It was further estimated that seven percent of all hang glider flights ended either in injury or fatality. In 1973, glider plane pilots numbered 13,395; and from 1960 through 1973, seventy-three deaths occurred in glider plane flying. Sport parachuting has drawn over forty thousand people, with ten to twelve fatal jumps being made each year. Another report documents the fact that when sky divers had jumped three or more years, seventy-one percent sustained injury.[149] It has been submitted that actions that are habituated and whose cumulative probability makes it very likely that the individual undertaking them will die as a consequence could be considered properly as suicidal.[150]

Society both encourages and promotes these types of "athletic" destructive behaviors. Why are some exercises of rational self-determination allowed and sanctioned (even encouraged for the en-ncement of local and state revenues) and others not? It has been suggested that the sport affiliated behaviors provide a type of "psychological service" to society in that those participating in various media-hyped high risk sports fulfill psychological needs for the viewing spectators.[151] Not only may a spectator participate vicariously with the actual participant but actually "defy, or even experience, death."[152]

> circus acts, whenever possible, it seems, are labeled "death-defying" to maximize their appeal to the public. This suggests that the greater the risk of death to the performer, the more the spectator is attracted to the event. A very daring but successful "defiance" of death may vicariously impart to the observer a feeling of elational well being, and even a momentary sense of immortality.[153]

Even though all these self-destructive behavioral actions have a high adverse economic effect on the public as to the maintenance and exten-sion of health care for those who pursue these high-risk or suicidal actions and sustain injuries therefrom, (many if not fatal, life-time incapacitating) little—if any—public effort has been launched to interfere blatantly or restrict these acts of self-endangerment. Only with the advent of the AIDS epidemic, have voices been raised suggesting a public quarantine of all known carriers of the disease in an effort to restrict its spread by promiscuous sexual conduct.[154] Surely if a large segment of modern society can be seen as viewing indirect self-destructive behaviors with ambivalence if not condonation, hope at least exists for direct forms of enlightened self-determination through what, traditionally, has been termed voluntary active euthanasia to be tolerated if not officially sanctioned in due course.

AIDING, ASSISTING, ABETTING OR ADVISING

The first do-it-yourself handbook on suicide, A GUIDE TO SELF-DELIVERANCE, was published in London by EXIT—The Society for the Right to Die with Dignity, a forty-five year old London based organization, during the Autumn of 1980.[155] Owing largely to a subse-quent judicial proceeding involving EXIT, this thirty-two page pam-phlet is now distributed to members of the organization, itself, of three months standing who are at least twenty-five years old.[156] Its basic aim is to assist the reader in dealing with the fear of non-existence or death and more particularly in overcoming the fear of the agony of dying.[157]

The pamphlet lists five different methods of suicide or self-deliverance under the headings: "Sedative Drugs and Plastic Bags;" "Drugs and Car Exhaust;" "Sedative Drugs and Hypothermia;" "Sedative Drugs and Drowning," and "Sedative Drugs Alone" (wherein appropriate dosages of various drugs and especially sedatives are listed).[158] The pamphlet counsels against acting in haste during periods of depression or loneliness and suggests consultation with Semaritans or family members.[159] Before making a final decision concerning self-deliverance, one is cautioned to consider the reasons for undertaking the act "over a substantial period of time" and whether the particular problems associated with the decision can be overcome by seeking medical or other help, or by changing life styles; and to be aware of the fact that no method of suicide provides a guarantee that the act will be achieved and, thus one could be left with a damaged brain or in worse physical condition than before the suicide was attempted.[160] Finally, consideration should be given to the fact that "of those who survive apparently serious suicide attempts, using methods which would normally have been expected to kill them, a significant proportion find that they can cope with life after all."[161] If things go awry, and there are snags in the suggested procedures, or if the information provided is found incorrect, the pamphlet reader is encouraged to report such matters to EXIT headquarters.[162]

As an organization, EXIT neither advocates nor does it express displeasure with suicide. It, rather, maintains a position of neutrality regarding such decisions as ones of personal belief or judgment.[163] By advocating a policy of rational self-deliverance, when freely chosen and appropriate, EXIT is careful to state that the act, itself, should not be taken as euphemistic. Self-deliverance

> implies that the person dies by his or her own hand, with a peaceful mind for reasons that those closest will endorse. They will know that they were not intended to feel guilt or grief, but rather share sympathetically in a final display of courage and good sense. No word to express the concept has existed until now ... since no one so far has made any effort to distinguish between the fulfillment of self-deliverance and the tragedy of other forms of suicide.[164]

Finally, as a socio-political organization, EXIT's objective is to work for the enactment into legislation of the previously defeated 1969 Voluntary Euthanasia Bill by Parliament. This Bill would authorize physicians to administer euthanasia to a patient when he had thirty days previously executed a written declaration to this effect in the presence of two witnesses. Two physicians—one of them a consultant—would bear the responsibility of certifying in writing that the at-risk patient would be—or is presently—suffering from a painful and incurable physical disease likely to cause severe states of distress and rendering the patient incapable of a rational existence. Ideally, the declaration would be executed well before the patient's good health declines and could be cancelled at any time. The waiting period of thirty days was designed to provide a type of built-in safeguard against what might be taken either as an impulsive or a reluctant decision.[165]

The Criminal Division of The Court of Appeal in London held on March 26, 1982—acting on an appeal from the Central Criminal Court against a conviction and sentence for conspiring and aiding and abetting suicide by Nicholas Reed, general secretary of EXIT—that Reed did not counsel or procure suicide with L (largely by and through publication and distribution of THE GUIDE TO SELF–DELIVERANCE.[166] Rather, Reed was properly convicted because he put L "in touch" with a potential suicide victim knowing full well that L would assist in the act of suicide if the situation so demanded and thus, then, either aid, abet, counsel or procure a suicide as prohibited by Statute and be properly convicted of conspiracy.[167] In reducing Reed's criminal sentence to eighteen months for the offense, the Court refused to accept the argument in mitigation that the agreement between L and Reed was only designed to promote a fuller understanding through counseling with individuals in stressful "at risk" situations, discouraging suicide when feasible or—depending upon an assessment of the most appropriate course of action—actively participating in its completion. The Court reasoned that regardless of the alternative or conditional nature of the agreement, the intention was still an obvious one to conspire to aid or abet a suicide.[168]

Mr. Justice Wolf in the case of *Attorney General v. Able and others*[169] ventured further into the thicket when the Attorney General sought to halt the distribution of the same pamphlet by applying in civil proceedings for a declaration that future supplies of the booklet to those who were known to be—or were likely to be—considering or intending to commit suicide constituted an offense under Section 2(1) of The Suicide Act of 1961, of aiding, abetting, counseling or procuring the suicide of another. Some eight thousand copies of the manual had been sold, on request, to members of EXIT twenty-five years and over and the increased popularity of the pamphlet over time was a cause of alarm to the

Attorney General. The civil action was maintained against the members of EXIT's executive committee, "who were respectable persons and who had issued the booklet out of genuine and strong held beliefs" rather than prosecute them criminally as a body.[170]

After reviewing the contents of the pamphlet at length, the Court refused the application for the declaration and concluded that while the distribution of the pamphlet could be an offense, before such a conclusion could be reached,

> .... it must at least be proved (a) that the alleged offender had the necessary intent, that is he intended that that person would be assisted by the booklet's contents, or otherwise encouraged to take or to attempt to take his own life; (b) that while he still had that intention, he distributed the booklet to such a person who read it; and (c) in addition, if an offense under S 2 of the 1961 Act is to be proved, that such a person was assisted or encouraged by so reading the booklet to take or attempt to take his own life, otherwise the alleged offender cannot be guilty of more than an attempt.[171]

Thus, it was held no offense under the Suicide Act of 1961 had been committed.[172]

As a result of the Suicide Act of 1961, not only was the crime of suicide abolished,[173] but also was the crime to attempt suicide.[174] But, interestingly, the Act does not entirely erase either the former religious prohibition of suicide as immoral nor disregard the Common Laws that held anyone who either incited or assisted another to commit suicide was himself guilty of abetting a crime "as a deduction from the supposed guilt of the deceased."[175] Even though this frame of reference is—under the Act—not permissible, the Suicide Act "in effect continues the old law by making it a statutory crime to aid, abet, counsel or procure a suicide or attempted suicide."[176] Yet, although the symbol or legacy of immorality still attaches to the Act's "on-record" validity, the actual practice of its enforcement is so light that but one or two prosecutions a year are made under it which, themselves, yield only a suspended sentence or probation.[177]

The social and religious standards that held, and in some cases still hold, suicide immoral prevent the law from dealing forthrightly with the dilemma and resolving it of allowing one to—legally—commit suicide, yet not be aided by another in completing the act.[178] This "old fashioned" manner of thinking that persists in devaluing enlightened acts of self-determination for perceived theological harmony of a cosmic nature, presents untold problems for incurably disabled but competent individuals who desperately need assistance in ending their travail with a semblance of dignity and compassion.

Two French authors, Claude Guillon and Yves le Bonniec, both members of the French Association for the Right to Die in Dignity, ADMD, co-authored a two hundred seventy-six page book entitled, SUICIDE: OPERATING INSTRUCTIONS, in April 1982.[179] Acclaimed as a best seller, the book aims to present a number of non-violent death alternatives "which do not degrade human dignity . . . by giving people the possibility of dying by methods less atrocious than the classic ones of razor blades, revolvers or hanging."[180] A prominent psychiatrist at a major Parisian hospital countered by stating, "Nine out of 10 people need help to be taught how to live, not how to die."[181]

In August, 1980, a former English journalist, Derek Humphrey, now living in Los Angeles, and fresh from his publishing successes with his 1978 book, JEAN'S WAY, (wherein he relates how he assisted his terminally ill wife in commiting suicide), helped organize HEMLOCK, an organization dedicated to supporting the right of terminally ill individuals to take their own lives.[182] LET ME DIE BEFORE I WAKE was authored by Mr. Humphrey in 1981 and is an effort to analyze case histories of terminally ill patients who sought successfully to end their lives. In the process of relating the successes, precise drug dose information is listed for any reader wishing to follow through themselves.[183] As a pro-choice society, HEMLOCK "does not encourage people to die: we encourage them to hang on for as long as possible; but "if for medical reasons life becomes unbearable, self-deliverance is a civil right that patients should have."[184]

In the United States, the First Amendment to the Constitution protects the "right to receive ideas,[185] even though the information received may disclose effective and painless ways of ending one's life.[186] The state may, however, restrict area of distribution and the manner of solicitation of such literature.[187] Although assisting suicide is still a crime in a number of states,[188] the power and force of the First Amendment is such that suicide manuals could not be suppressed[189]—even though there is a widespread concern among some that an unchecked distribution of these and other similar suicide manuals might put those individuals who are depressed or suicidal "over the brink."[190] In *Branderburg v. State of Ohio*,[191] in a concurring opinion, Mr. Justice Douglas summed up the central dilemma of First Amendment mandates and state interference by stating that,

> The line between what is permissible and not subject to control and what may be made impermissible are subject to regulation is the line between ideas and overt acts.[192]

In the *per curiam* of the Court, it was stated with clarity that the only reason for allowing an interference with free speech and the free press would be when the use of force or violation of the law, "is directed to inciting or producing imminent lawless action and is likely to incite or produce such action."[193] Obviously, the publication, sale and distribution of suicide manuals would not fall within the *Branderburg* exception because such a manual, of the type distributed by EXIT—for example—does not *advocate* "imminent lawless action" (since suicide has been decriminalized and assisted suicides are seldom prosecuted with vigor)[194] of a violent nature. A mere publication does not strike a chord of immediacy since a "once over" perusal would not normally produce or give rise to precipitous action; rather reflection upon it, as well as other sources, would be consulted over time.[195]

Even though state legislation, as observed, prohibits assisting another in his acts of suicide,[196] and is theoretically prosecutable under general homicide statutes,[197] in fact the enforcement and prosecution of these acts is negligible.[198] Yet, again, in theory these acts of assistance could be classified as involuntary manslaughter,[199] coercion,[200] general recklessness,[201] or criminal negligence.[202] As to the issue of remoteness of actions imposing liability, the Model Penal Code requires the actual result to involve a kind of harm or injury that is *not remote* or accidental,[203] or—if reckless or negligently induced—"not within the risk of what the actor is aware, or in the case of negligence, of which he should be aware."[204]

> What will usually turn on the determination [of whether the defendant caused the result] will not be the criminality of defendant's conduct but rather the gravity of his offense. Since the actor, by hypothesis, has sought to cause a criminal result, or has been reckless or negligent with respect to such a result, he will be guilty of some crime under a well-considered penal code even if he is not held for the actual result; i.e., he will be guilty of attempt, assault, or some offense involving risk creation. . . . Thus the issue in penal law is very different than in torts. Only in form is it, in penal law, a question of the actor's liability. In substance, it is a question of the severity of sentence which the Court is authorized or obliged to impose.[205]

Designing a Resolution

The concept of assisted rational suicide, rational suicide or the right of the terminally ill patients to take their own life, is being accepted more and more by both the legal and medical professions.[206] One prominent Los Angeles attorney has observed that state laws which classify attempted suicide as a crime have been eliminated for the most part and that there is a growing movement to reform the laws against aiding or abetting suicide.[207]

Because of the plethora of complex moral and ethical questions raised under suicide assistance laws, prosecutors are reluctant, generally, to bring strong actions under them.[208] A member of the New York County District Attorney's office in Manhattan observed that a case-by-case method is used to evaluate suicide incidents brought under specific state laws prohibiting either aiding or abetting suicide.[209] He stated that, "Incidents in which persons may have questionable motives such as familial gain, for encouraging or assisting another person's suicide . . . are the type of case we'd be likely to prosecute."[210] He continued by noting that in those cases involving terminally ill patients prosecutions is less likely to be maintained simply because the courts are recording reluctance, "to convict defendants when the moral issues of mercy and the patient's privacy rights are involved."[211]

A former Chairman of the American Medical Association's Ad Hoc Council on Medical Ethics acknowledged recently that a physician must recognize that after advising a patient regarding the prognosis of his disease, the patient—himself—has a right to decide what course of treatment will follow or, for that matter, to choose suicide.[212] Perhaps somewhat overstating the matter, he concluded, "The day of paternalism of the profession is long since gone."[213]

The compelling state interest to prevent assisted suicide is quite weak when the act is undertaken because of a terminal or severely handicapping illness, but admittedly more tenable when a decision to undertake suicide is made when death is not imminent. The state has persuasive arguments to see that its citizens remain healthy, care for their dependents and honor their contracts to fulfill binding legal obligations.[214] Yet, the most humane and practical manner in which to deal with the immediate conundrum is to have suicide and aiding and abetting its execution defined statutorily as non criminal.[215]

The purpose of such model legislation would be to allow the state to withdraw from its intrusive forays into the basic liberties of its competent, but incapacitated and terminally ill citizens, who wish to follow a course of enlightened self-determination and thereby end their lives. Such a uniform legislative declaration would—ideally—allow those lacking capacity, owing to infancy, mental incompetence or unconsciousness, to utilize the protections of surrogate decision making and exercise the same liberty as their competent fellow citizens.

More directly regarding the competent decision maker here, the states should enact legislation making it lawful for any individual to furnish another equally competent individual "with the means to commit suicide so long as the person committing suicide takes the last definite step to initiate the suicidal act."[216] Under such a legislative design, not only a physician—but anyone for that matter—would be allowed to make available to the individual desiring suicide the means to effectuate the act. In the absence of coercion, the competence of the individual committing the suicide would likely need to be recognized as a defense against civil liability for those assisting with the act, itself. A mandatory witness declaration prior to an assisted suicide might well be considered as an additional precaution against foul play "masquerading as an assisted suicide."[217]

Absent a bold and imaginative legislative plan of action among the states, it will remain for the courts to be brought more and more into the deliberative decision making process here and thereby intrude not only into the confidentiality of the doctor-patient relationship, patient autonomy, but familial privacy and independence as well.[218]

SUICIDE PREVENTION AND MANAGEMENT

One line of reasoning holds that an act of suicide can never be "chosen" since overwhelming compulsions make a free choice at best nugatory—if not totally void.[219] Accordingly, "no human being, no matter how determined he or she may seem to be to put an end to life, does not somewhere cherish the hope of being saved."[220] Thus, the aim of suicide prevention and management is directed not so much toward the achievement of a reduction in suicide rates as it is to helping distressed "at risk" individuals find an avenue of self-realization and human dignity rather than of failure.[221] And beyond this simple purpose, suicide prevention can be seen as transcending itself into "courageous humaneness" where—in efforts to implement the goals of a prevention program—men and women of convictions come together in a sincere effort to serve others and seek to "implement humane thinking."[222] In essence, what suicide prevention is all about is—in a word—"crisis intervention."[223]

Counseling and professional psychiatric therapy form the cornerstones of an effective suicide prevention program.[224] Poison detoxification centers and convalescent centers (particularly for alcoholics) and follow-up care are also utilized.[225] Without question, the most effective lay program was started in 1953 in London by an Anglican priest who simply used the telephone as a medium of communication with despondent, friendless people who contemplated suicide.[226] Catapulted into public awareness by radio, television and press coverage, the organization— called the Samaritans—has grown and become more professional as well as more successful than ever before imagined.[227]

The underlying concept or principle of the success of The Samaritans is that of "beneficiary" defined—simply—as "the offering of friendship by ordinary people to ordinary people, with no strings attached."[228] The befriender expects neither material reward of any nature nor gratitude for his work. Should the client wish to unburden himself, the befriender listens as a friend, and may introduce him to a new circle of friends.[229] The reintegration of anomic people into society is one of the befriender's primary tasks."[230] The extent of the period of befriendment can be short or long termed. For example, helping an acute reactive depressive through one crisis period would give rise to a relatively short period of befriending, while dealing with a schizophrenic might well extend over a period of time. In order to prevent an emotional attachment or involvement by the initially untrained befriender with a client, a closely supervised training program has been structured that places absolute control with each Branch Director of a Samaritan Chapter.[231] In a word, then, it can be seen that the Samaritans take a totally advisory—as opposed to directoral—approach to their work.[232]

Interestingly, by rendering the service of advice, oftentimes one may cure another's problem during the course of advising.

> Loneliness and the absence of human affection are states which exacerbate many other problems; disappointment, reduction to poverty, etc., seem less impossible to bear in the presence of the affection of another. Hence simply to be a friend, or to find someone a friend, may be the largest contribution one can make either to helping a person be rational or see clearly what is rational for him to do; this service may make

one who was contemplating suicide feel that there is now a future for him which is possible to face.[233]

Organized efforts directed toward suicide prevention began at the turn of the century.[234] Perhaps the very first such organization, the Lemberger *Freiwilligen Rettungsgesellschaft* (The Lemberg Volunteer Rescue Society) existed from 1893 to 1906 in Germany and served as a volunteer emergency service designed to aid not only suicide and attempted suicide cases, but provide other types of emergency service.[235] A counterpart organization was also found in Budapest, Hungary.[236]

The aftermath of World War 1 that witnessed widespread hunger and financial chaos throughout Europe, also was the setting for the development of a movement to operate specially designed preventive clinics to cope with the *Lebensmüdden* in Vienna.[237] The outpouring from people who asked to be protected from their "own desperate thoughts" was significant.[238] Indeed, one distinguished commentator noted that, "Token human contact could prevent the fatal act in ninety percent of the cases" of suicide.[239]

In the United States, it was not until after World War II that suicide prevention centers were started.[240] Indeed, in 1958, the first publicly supported suicide prevention center organized to deal "with the important other-than-purely-medical aspects of individual suicide attempts" was funded by the United States Public Health Service and administered by The University of Southern California in the Los Angeles community.[241]

Today, a vast network of counseling services are offered by various church and volunteer organizations.[242] The National Institute of Mental Health has been successful in showing suicide to be both a health and a social problem and—at the same time—instilling a commitment on the part of mental health leaders to better understand and thereby hopefully control it.[243] Yet, if this commitment is to be realized totally instead of being but a vacuous "pipe dream," a sound financial basis must be established nationally to support the suicide prevention centers other than through volunteer and church supporting projects. Ideally, this effort at suicide prevention should be assumed by local communities and placed as an integral part or line item in their annual budgets—much in the same manner in which financial support is budgeted for local health department mental health clinics and other governmental agency budgets. Indeed, in an effort to provide continuity of operation, in the future, suicide prevention centers will likely maintain themselves and function through comprehensive mental health clinics.[244]

Involuntary Psychiatric Commitments

Although the criminal laws in some states allow suicides and attempted suicides to be punished, in actuality, violations under them are infrequent.[245] Yet, for persons believed to be suicidal, civil commitment procedures still enjoy support.[246] For those considered mentally ill, dangerous to themselves or in need of either care or treatment, state mental health laws authorize both long-term commitment by way of hospitalization or institutionalization.[247] State legislation also allows for emergency detention in order to prevent suicide.[248]

Most commitment statutes that exercise a form of benevolent coercion designed as such to prevent self-injury by suicide, do not only specify that the defendant must be viewed as dangerous to himself if *not* committed, but that he is also adjudged mentally ill; and occasionally a statutory specification directs the dangerousness be a *consequence* of the mental illness.[249] All too often today questions concerning mental illness are decided on the basis of physicians using standard psychiatric classifications which they are uncertain and ill-at-ease in applying, personal moral judgment of the lifestyles of the defendants or even lay notions of mental health.[250] Complex questions of causation are not considered or confusingly applied since the working assumption made is "that dangerousness and mental illness imply one another.[251]

The argument that suicide is harmful must be rejected out and out as specious; for nothing concrete is known of the fate that befalls one who takes his own life. Practically, it is surely within the realm of imagination to posture a case where suicide could well be recognized as the lesser of two evils—as where one commits the act in order either to escape excruciating pain or be relieved of a terminal illness. Case histories of suicide also show a more willing condonation or acceptance of suicides precipitated in order to prevent enemies of the state from obtaining national secrets through use of torture, to end a desolate and tedious life, to preserve personal or family honor (or reputation) pending a scandal or to publicize a grave personal, group or political injustice.[252]

Other case studies reveal the fact that an act of suicide may appear—to the outside viewer—in clear disproportion to what is viewed as the precipitating cause.[253] Numerous attempts at suicide which are rooted in deep guilt feelings over social experiences and which, to others, seem insignificant, would comprise one such clear paradigm. It is quite difficult to remember distress is *subjective*. Thus, although a non-participant may view a stress engendering situation as within the parameters of tolerable distress, this in no way may serve to mitigate the real anguish of the individual who—feeling life intolerable—ends it himself by suicide.[254]

Owing to a basic misunderstanding, then, of the personal circumstances that give rise to each suicide and a common tendency to project one's health or well-adjusted attitude to a life situation, and thereby being unable to relate to a suicide, society concludes that suicide is undesirable; it is furthermore both unchristian and atheistic since absolute despair is totally inconsistent with faith in God.[255] Again, "if one is coping well and observes that most others cope well, one may not be able to understand the behavior of those not coping well."[256] Thus in learning of suicides, the conclusion is made inevitably by the average ordinary "reasonable" person that the act is always to be viewed as totally irrational and, indeed, undesirable.[257]

Preventing suicides means someone else is making a decision that a potential suicide attempter is better off alive and suffering than dead.[258] The right to die or but exercise ultimate autonomy is other words—best viewed as but a co-ordinate or extension of the right to live with dignity—is but a hollow concept or principle if it can only be exercised when it is thought to be consistent with what others regard as reasonable or appropriate.[259] "While it may seem anomalous to speak of a 'right to die,' the infringement of this right seriously jeopardizes the right to live one's life as one wishes, and not to live it when it is no longer possible to do so as one wishes."[260]

There is much current debate over the scope and need for involuntary civil commitment and—more specifically—whether the state should seek to use its coercive powers to deprive those with mental illness of their liberty or whether involuntary civil commitment should be abolished totally in favor of other systems of social action. How laws should define, delegate and control state action exercised under a broad police power or an equally broad power of *parens patriae* is also of concern.[261]

This debate has intensified over the past twenty years both in the courts and state legislatures,[262] and resulted in not only the recognition of a number of procedural rights for individuals who are subjected to proceedings for commitment (including prior notice, an opportunity to be heard, the right to counsel, and the right to judicial review of an

initial commitment order)[263] but the development of substantive commitment criteria (a determination of mental illness and that one is dangerous to self and others)[264] and a requirement for the least restrictive
alternative disposition—or least drastic method of treatment be provided.[265] These developments have been regarded as raising serious
barriers to efforts designed to offer effective treatment opportunities to
those in need of them.[266]

A growing number of states have restricted, legislatively, their authority to force treatment upon the mentally ill.[267] This is all in keeping
with a national trend toward deinstitutionalization of mental patients.[268]
Community health systems now provide out patient psychiatric care
as a viable alternative to confinement. Indeed, as a consequence of
significant and varied litigative success concerning deinstitutionalization and involuntary commitment, a constitutional requirement has
been structured mandating treatment be provided in the least restrictive
environment.[269]

Yet, a trend is but a trend—and certainly not a uniform response. The
present system of involuntary commitment is tied to hospitalization and
fails to embrace current state of the art therapeutic alternative.[270] Whether
all forms of involuntary therapy should be abolished is a vexatious
question to be sure.[271] But—consistent with basic concepts of autonomy
and self-determination, and the *parens patriae* power of the state—reform
could be undertaken by a greater utilization of the laws of guardianship
that would empower duly appointed guardians to authorize treatment
for obviously incapacitated or at-risk individuals.[272] This could, in turn,
promote a system where involuntary treatment of those bereft of rational
powers of discernment while requiring treatment, would nonetheless
receive their therapy in the least restrictive setting—with confinement to
a hospital being used only as a last resort.[273]

Today, a general movement is being charted among state legislatures
that de-emphasizes a stated concern for an individual's treatment needs
and—instead—places concern for evaluating and containing the level of
dangerousness of the afflicted individual.[274] It is to be acknowledged that
an exercise of state power directed toward the prevention of harm to
others is an inherent police power, just as state enforced treatment is an
exercise of the *parens patriae* power.[275] Obviously, efforts designed to
prevent harm to one's self treat of both a police power and a *parens patriae*
power.[276] "The revisions of civil commitment law in the direction of a

single standard of dangerousness therefore reflect a determination that *parens patriae* standing alone is an insufficient basis for commitment of the incompetent mentally ill."[277] It has been suggested that the overriding need for treatment of mentally imbalanced individuals could be met by recognizing a standard that permitted commitment for one who "is mentally ill and in need of care or treatment in a mental hospital but because of illness lacks sufficient insight or capacity to make a rational decision concerning treatment."[278] The long term testing value of this standard has yet to be determined and verified. Nonetheless, the application of the criterion to the commitment process has an unquestioned and equally far-reaching impact on the rights of the patient while hospitalized and especially his ability or his "right" to refuse treatment.[279]

Other Mechanisms—The Ulysses Contract

The voluntary commitment contract, denominated the Ulysses Contract, provides a means for giving advance consent to treatment for a mental disorder and incorporates a *waiver* of the right to refuse treatment when administered subsequently.[280] As Ulysses instructed his crew to restrain him before they sailed through the island waters of the Sirens—and to ignore all requests that he might make for release during the passage—individuals executing a Ulysses Contract would be bargaining with their physicians to disregard those instructions that might issue during a relapse (as for example refusing needed treatment) for a limited period of time.[281] The simile could also be expanded by choosing—in the alternative—to recognize the state as the crew servicing Ulysses, seeking, as such, to restrain those unwilling to protect themselves from harm.[282]

Underlying the efficacy of the Ulysses Contract is personal autonomy or what has been termed "the principle of self-paternalism."[283] Undergirding this principle is the inherent recognition that every person has a true identity that acts, in the long run, to maximize his best interests.[284] Accordingly, although one's desires, interests and attitudes will over time vary, the decisions of the true identity should always be recognized and maintained over contrary expressions.[285] If implementing legislation could be passed, codifying the concepts of the Ulysses Contract, the contract would furnish an important construct through which the state could seek to enforce those rational wishes of one's true identity.[286]

Model Laws

Under a proposed Model State Commitment Statute authored by the American Psychiatric Association,[287] the state's *parens patriae* power is given significant weight and forms the basis for the involuntary emergency admission of an individual for both evaluation and treatment—if necessary—when a determination is made that he is suffering from a severe mental disorder that prevents informed decision making regarding treatment and is thus *likely* to suffer substantial mental deterioration or physical deterioration or *likely* harm others.[288] Under the provisions of the statute, an additional thirty day period of commitment is authorized if a judicial determination is made that the individual at-risk is *likely* to suffer severe mental deterioration if treatment is not continued.[289]

This model statute would mandate treatment for the incapacitated individual unable to make rational treatment decisions and stress the fact that treatment, itself, is the central basis or justification for civil commitment.[290] In some respects, the model statute criteria "are broader than those in some current state laws (for example in providing for commitment of persons whose mental state is likely to deteriorate), while in other respects the criteria are stricter (for example in permitting commitment only of persons who lack capacity)."[291] It is thought, "that relatively few persons who would now be committable as dangerous would not be committable under the Model Law, and that many severely disordered people who are now committable as gravely disordered could be committed under the Model Law."[292]

ENDNOTES

1. SUICIDOLOGY: CONTEMPORARY DEVELOPMENTS 6 (E. SHNEIDMAN ed. 976).
2. Id.
3. Id. at 7.

It has been suggested that the first known document dealing specifically with suicide is to be found in DISPUTE OVER SUICIDE—an Egyptian writing thought to be from either the Middle Kingdom or earlier, around 2100 B.C. Bearing some marked similarities to the Book of Job, it focuses on a debate a man has with his soul, prompted as such, because of a series of misfortunes that have befallen him. The debate explores the values of holding onto life and seeking new pleasures or ending it and its present level of suffering. Thus, what is seen—then—is that so long as written accounts of history have been kept, suicide has been recorded. D. de Cantanzo, SUICIDE AND SELF DAMAGING BEHAVIOUR 26 (1984).

4. Supra note 1 at 7.

See generally, Daube, The Linguistics of Suicide, 1 PHIL. & PUB. AFFAIRS 4 (1972).

5. See E. Durkheim, SUICIDE: STUDY IN SOCIOLOGY (J. SPAULDING, G. SIMPSON transl. 1952).

6. A. TOYNBEE, et al, MAN'S CONCERN WITH DEATH 264 (1968).

7. M. HEIFETZ, THE RIGHT TO DIE 73 (1975).

8. E. DURKHEIM; A STUDY IN SOCIOLOGY 341 (J. SPAULDING, G. SIMPSON transl. 1952).

9. Id.

10. Id. at 13.

The most accepted psychoanalytic view of suicide is that it is a form of displacement or a desire to kill someone who has thwarted the individual suicidee. Id. at 24. Today, however, suicidologists hold the opinion that hostility, frustrated dependency, hopelessness and helplessness also have considerable significance in promoting suicide. SUICIDOLOGY: CONTEMPORARY DEVELOPMENTS 10 (E. SHNEIDMAN ed. 1976).

11. Supra note 8 at 326.

12. SUICIDE: THE PHILOSOPHICAL ISSUES 2 (M. BATTIN, D. MAYO eds. 1980).

13. Id.

14. Id.

15. Id.

16. Hankoff, Judaic Origins of the Suicide Prohibitions in SUICIDE THEORY AND CLINICAL ASPECTS Ch. 1 (L. Hankoff, B. Einsidler eds. 1979); Feberow, Cultural History of Suicide in SUICIDE IN DIFFERENT CULTURES 1, 3–4 (N. Farberow ed. 1975); A. ALVAREZ, THE SAVAGE GOD 41–63 (1971); Smart, Death in the Judaeo-Christian Tradition in MAN'S CONCERN WITH DEATH at 116 *passim* (A. TOYNBEE, et al eds. 1968).

17. Id.

18. See, JUDGES 9:54; JUDGES 16:30; 1 SAMUEL 31:4; 2 SAMUEL 17:23; 1 KINGS 16:18; 2 MACCABEES 7:1–42; 2 MACCABEES 10:113 and 2 MACCABEES 14:41.

19. D. de Cantanzo, SUICIDE AND SELF DAMAGING BEHAVIOUR 27 (1984); N. St. John-Stevas, THE RIGHT TO LIFE 58 (1964).

Perhaps the most notable exception to this position was when some nine hundred sixty Jews at Massada in 73 A.D. committed acts of mass suicide in order to avoid an inevitable capture by victorious Romans. de Cantanzo at 27. See Hankoff, supra note 16.

20. Amundsen, The Physicians Obligation to Prolong Life: A Medical Duty Without Classical Roots, 8 HASTINGS CENTER RPT. 23, 26–27 (Aug. 1978).

21. Farberow, Cultural History of Suicide in SUICIDE IN DIFFERENT CULTURES 1, 6 (N. Faberow ed. 1975).

22. Amundsen, supra note 20.

See Daube, The Linguistics of Suicide, 1 PHIL. & PUB. AFFAIRS 387 (1972).

23. Id.

Shintoism, Budhism and Hinduism allow suicide in case of incurable disease, while the Islamic and Judaic religions condemn it and Catholicism opposes it. M. HEIFETZ, THE RIGHT TO DIE 78 (1975).

24. SUICIDE: THE PHILOSOPHICAL ISSUES 2 (M. Battin, D. Mayo eds. 1980).

25. W. DURANT, THE STORY OF CIVILIZATION: THE LIFE OF GREECE 655–657 (1939).

26. A. ALVAREZ, THE SAVAGE GOD 58–67 (1972).

27. Id. at 18.

28. Supra note 25 at 657.

29. G. WILLIAMS, THE SANCTITY OF LIFE AND THE CRIMINAL LAW 252 (1972).

30. See DeLacy, Epicureanism and The Epicurean School, 3 ENCYCLOPEDIA OF PHILOSOPHY 2 (P. EDWARDS ed. 1067).

31. See Hallie, Stoicism, 8 ENCYCLOPEDIA OF PHILOSOPHY 19–22 (P. EDWARDS ed. 1967).

32. Id.

33. G. WILLIAMS, THE SANCTITY OF LIFE AND THE CRIMINAL LAW 21 (1972). See Hudson, Suicide: Madness or The Noble Roman Way?, THE PHAROS 45 (Fall 1952).

34. Id.

35. Id.

36. Id.

37. Id.

38. Williams, supra at 33.

39. D. PORTWOOD, COMMON SENSE SUICIDE 22 (1978); G. WILLIAMS, THE SANCTITY OF LIFE AND THE CRIMINAL LAW 254–255 (1972).

40. M. HEIFETZ, THE RIGHT TO DIE 77 (1975).

Actually, in 452, the Council of Arles declared suicide a crime and concluded that it was caused "by a diabolically inspired fury." E. DURKHEIM, SUICIDE: A STUDY IN SOCIOLOGY 327 (J. Spaulding, G. Simpson transl. 1952).

It was not until 563, however, that a penal sanction was first imposed at the Council of Prague. Accordingly, the victims of suicide were disallowed a burial mass "and the singing of psalms" as their bodies were buried. Civil penalties were added subsequently. DURKHEIM, Id.

In tenth century England, suicides were associated with robbers, assassins and all other criminals and it was customary to drag the body of the suicide — pierced with a stick crossways — through the streets and bury it on a highway. In Zurich, if a suicide stabbed himself, a fragment of the wood in which the knife was fixed was driven into the body near the head. Similarly, if he had drowned himself, he was then buried under five feet of water in the sand. Durkheim, at 328.

41. P. & L. LANDSBERG, THE EXPERIENCE OF DEATH AND THE MODEL PROBLEM OF SUICIDES 77 *passim* (1953).

42. In Book I of The City of God, Augustine stated: "It is not without significance,

that in no passage of the holy canonical books there can be found either divine precept or permission to take away our own life, whether for the sake of entering the enjoyment of immortality, or of shunning, or ridding ourselves of anything whatsoever." W. OATES, BASIC WRITINGS OF ST. AUGUSTINE 27 (1948).

43. Id. at 28, 32–33.

44. Id.

45. See T. Aquinas, SUMMA THEOLOGICA 1470 (Dominican ed. 1947).

The reason for the sinfulness of the act was tied to three arguments: it contradicted the natural inclination toward self-preservation and charity, it inflicted injury upon the particular community wherein the suicidee lived and it violated the exercise of God's rights as Creator over man's destiny. Id.

46. Marzen, O'Dowd, Crone & Balch, Suicide: A Constitutional Right? 24 DUQ. L. REV. 1, 31 *passim* (1985).

47. Id. at 33.

48. Id.

49. Id. at 34.

50. Id. at 35.

51. Id.

52. Id. at 36.

53. Id. at 37, quoting Kant, Metaphysics of Morals in METAPHYSICAL PRIN-CIPLES OF VIRTUES 83 (Elington trans. 1964).

54. Id., quoting Kant, Metaphysics of Morals in METAPHYSICAL PRINCIPLES OF VIRTUE 83–84 (Elington trans. 1964); 1 Kant, LECTURES ON ETHICS 152 (L. Infield, trans. 1963).

55. Regina v. Doody, 6 Cox Crim. Cas. 463 (1854).

See also, Regina v. Burgess 168 ENG. REP. 1387 (1862); Regina v. Man, 2 K.B. 107 (1914).

56. G. WILLIAMS, THE SANCTITY OF LIFE, Ch. 2 (1957).

57. 4 Blackstone, COMMENTARIES Ch. 14 at 189, 190 (1857).

See generally, Silving, Suicide and Law in CLUES TO SUICIDE, Ch. 9 (E. Shneidman, N. Farberow eds. 1957).

58. The Forfeiture Act of 1870, 33 & 34 VICT. c. 23.

59. The Suicide Act of 1961, 9 & 10 Eliz. 2, c. 60.

60. Id.

61. Marzen, O'Dowd, Crone & Balch, Suicide: A Constitutional Right? 24 DUQ. L. REV. 1, 100 (1985).

62. Id. at 63, 64.

63. Id. at 98, 99.

Yet, there is judicial precedent in the states of Alabama, Oregon and South Carolina that holds suicide to be a crime. See, *Southern Life & Health Ins. Co. v. Wynn*, 29 Ala. App. 209, 194 So. 421 (1940); *Wycoff v. Mutual Life Ins. Co.*, 173 Or. 592, 147 P.2d 227 (1944); *State v. Levell*, 13 S.E. 319, (S.C. 1891).

64. ALASKA STAT. §§ 11.41.1-(a) (2), 11.41.120 (a) (2) (1983); ARIZ. REV. STAT. ANN. § 13-1103 (A) (3) (Supp. 1985); ARK. STAT. ANN. § 41-1504 (1) (1977); CAL. PENAL CODE § 401 (West 1970); COLO. REV. STAT. § 18-3-104 (1) (b) (1978);

CONN. GEN. STAT. § 53a-56 (a) (2) (West 1972); DEL. CODE ANN. tit. 11, § 645 (1979); FLA. STAT. ANN. § 782.08 (West 1976); KAN. STAT. ANN. § 21-3406 (1974); ME. REV. STAT. ANN. tit. 17A, § 204 comment (1983); MINN. STAT. ANN. § 609.215 (West 1964); MISS. CODE ANN. § 41-21-61 (d), -73 (4) (Supp. 1984); MONT. CODE ANN. § 45-5-105 (1983); NEB. REV. STAT. § 28-307 (1979); N.J. STAT. ANN. § 2C:11-6 (West 1982); N.M. STAT. ANN. § 40A-2-5 (1953), § 30-2-4 (1984); N.Y. PENAL LAW §§ 120.35, 125.15 (3) (McKinney 1975); OKLA. STAT. ANN. tit. 21 § 813 (West 1983); ORE. REV. STAT. §§ 163.117, 163.125 (1) (b) (Repl. 1983); 18 PA. CONS. STAT. ANN. § 2505 (Purdon 1983); P.R. LAWS ANN. tit. 33, § 1385 (1956); S.C. CODE ANN. § 16-1-10 (Law Co-op 1976); S.D. CODE §§ 13.1902 (1968); TEX. PENAL CODE § 22.09 (Vernon 1974); REV. WASH. CODE §§ 9A92.010 (213-17) (1977); WIS. STAT. ANN. § 940.12 (West 1982).

   See also Englehardt & Malloy, Suicide and Assisting Suicide: A Critique of Legal Sanctions, 36 So. W. L. J. 1003, 1020 n's 69, 70, for various case authorities holding to the same effect as these statutes.

   65. *Burnett v. People*, 204 Ill. 208, 68 N.E. 505 (1903); *People v. Roberts*, 211 Mich. 187, 198, 178 N.E. 690, 693; *Blackburn v. State*, 23 Ohio St. 146, 162–63 (1870).

   66. Note, Criminal Liability of Participants in Suicide: *State v. Williams*, 5 MD. L. REV. 324 (1941).

   67. Id.

   68. *Commonwealth v. Dennis*, 105 Mass. 162 (1870).

   69. Brenner, Undue Influence in the Criminal Law: A Proposed Analysis of the Criminal Offense Causing Suicide, 47 ALB. L. REV. 62 (1982).

   70. D.C. CODE ANN. § 6-2428 (Supp. 1984).

   71. W. VA. CODE § 16-30-8 (a) (1984).

   72. See A. SCOTT, CRIMINAL LAWS IN COLONIAL VIRGINIA 27 (1930).

   73. See e.g., *State v. Alley*, 594 S. W. 2d 832 (Tenn. 1980).

   74. HAWAII REV. STAT. § 707-702 (1) (b) (1976).

   75. IND. CODE ANN. § 35-42-1-2 (West 1978).

   76. State v. Campbell 217 IOWA 848, 251 N.W. 717 (1933); KY. REV. STAT. § 500.020 (1985); *Oubre v. Mutual Life Ins. Co. of New York*, 21 SO. 2d 191 (La. Ct. App. 1945); NEV. STAT. §§ 458, 667 (1967); N.C. GEN. STAT. § 14-17.1 (1981); N.D. SESS. LAWS 215, 300 (1973); UTAH CODE ANN. § 76-1-105 (1978); WYO. STAT. ANN. § 6-1-102 (Supp. 1985).

   77. Survey, Euthanasia: Criminal, Tort, Constitutional and Legislative Considerations, 48 NOTRE DAME L. REV. 1202, 1206 (1973).

   See also, W. LaFave & A. Scott, Jr., CRIMINAL LAW 569 (1972).

   78. Marzen, O'Dowd, Crone & Balch, Suicide: A Constitutional Right? 24 DUQ. L. REV. 1, 98 (1985).

   See also, Schulman, Suicide and Suicide Prevention: A Legal Analysis, 54 A.B.A.J. 855, 858–860 (1968); Shaffer, Legal Views of Suicide, in SUICIDOLOGY: CONTEMPORARY DEVELOPMENTS, Ch. 13 (E. Shneidman ed. 1976).

   79. P. ARIES, WESTERN ATTITUDES TOWARDS DEATH: FROM THE MIDDLE AGES TO PRESENT, Ch. 1, (P. Ranum trans. 1974).

   80. Id., Ch. 2.

81. Id.

82. Id.

83. Id., Chs. 3, 4.

84. C. BECKER, THE HEAVENLY CITY OF THE PHILOSOPHERS 148–149 (1932).

85. Id. See also, A. ALVAREZ, The Savage God 41 *passim* (1971) for a history of death practices.

86. Toynbee, Changing Attitudes Towards Death in the Modern Western World in MAN'S CONCERN WITH DEATH at 122 (A. Toynbee, et al eds. 1968).

87. Id.

88. Id. at 131.

See generally, J. MITFORD, THE AMERICAN WAY OF DEATH (1963).

89. G. SMITH, MEDICAL–LEGAL ASPECTS OF CRYONICS: PROSPECTS FOR IMMORTALITY (1983); Smith, Cryonic Suspension and The Law, 17 OMEGA 1 (1986–87); Smith, The Iceperson Cometh: Cryonics and The Law, 1 J. CONTEMP. HEALTH ISSUES 23 (1983).

90. Toynbee, Changing Attitudes Towards Death in the Modern Western World in MAN'S CONCERN WITH DEATH at 131 (A. Toynbee et al eds. 1968).

91. Id.

See generally, Society for the Right to Die, THE PHYSICIANS AND THE HOPELESSLY ILL PATIENT 5 *passim* (1985).

92. Will, In Praise of Mortality in THE MORNING AFTER: AMERICAN SUCCESSES AND EXCESSES 410 at 411, 412 (G. Will ed. 1986).

93. J. Meerloo, SUICIDE AND MASS SUICIDE 111 (1962).

94. D. MAGUIRE, DEATH BY CHOICE 216, 217 (1975).

95. Id.

96. Id.

97. Id.

98. Id.

99. Id.

100. Id. at 217.

101. Id.

102. Fox, The Recent Decline of Suicide in Britain: The Role of The Samaritan Suicide Prevention Movement in Britain, in SUICIDOLOGY: CONTEMPORARY DEVELOPMENTS at 501, 502 (E. Schneidman ed. 1976).

103. Id. at 502.

104. Id.

See AIDS Patients Found at Higher Risk of Suicide: Treatment Urged for Depression, Delirium Associated with Illness, Wash. Post, Mar. 4, 1988, at A5, col. 1.

105. Peck, Towards a Theory of Suicide: The Case for Modern Fatalism 11 OMEGA 1 (1980–81).

106. R. LIFTON, THE BROKEN CONNECTION 256, 257 (1979).

107. D. de Cantanzo, SUICIDE AND SELF DAMAGING BEHAVIOUR Ch. 13 at 158, 159 *passim* (1981).

108. J. JACOBS, ADOLESCENT SUICIDE Ch. 1 (1970); E. DURKHEIM, SUICIDE: A STUDY IN SOCIOLOGY 10 (1951).

109. Durkheim, supra.

110. J. MEERLOO, SUICIDE AND MASS SUICIDE 65 (1962).

111. Id. at 2, 20.

112. Id. at 21.

The use of hunger strikes, that all too often end in death, as a form of social and political bargaining power, have come into greater focus as a consequence of the volatile situations in Northern Ireland. The Roman Catholic Church finds a growing reluctance to judge someone who commits suicide in this manner and to deny them a proper church burial. Briggs, Catholic Church Endeavors to Put Hunger Strikes in Perspective, N.Y. TIMES, June 8, 1981, at B1, col. 1.

113. Hudgens, Preventing Suicide, 308 NEW ENG. J. MED. 897 (April 14, 1983).

See also, E. ROBBINS, THE FINAL MONTHS 12 (1981).

In a clinical analysis of the motivations for suicide in over one thousand cases, it was found that: nearly ten percent of the suicides were not motivated consciously, but were—rather—impulsive acts committed by either deranged or alcoholics; twenty-five percent were committed by people regarded as mentally unstable; forty percent acted on the basis of impulse arising from a strong emotion (pain, distress, shame, defeat) yet are not viewed as psychotic; and twenty-five percent undertake suicide after a thorough consideration of the pros and cons of life and death. J. MEERLOO, SUICIDE AND MASS SUICIDE 25 (1962).

114. Hudgens, supra.

115. Id.

116. Boyd, The Increasing Rate of Suicide by Firearm, 308 NEW ENG. J. MED. 872 (1983).

117. Hudgens, supra note 113 at 898.

118. Streitfeld, Suicide in Pairs: Together in Final Anguish, WASH. POST, Mar. 5, 1987, at B5, col. 1.

119. Id.

See Mitchell, What Love is About, as They Lay Dying, WASH. POST, Sept. 6, 1985, at D2, col. 1.

120. Id.

121. Id.

122. Id.

123. Id.

124. Id.

125. Id.

126. Id.

127. Carlson, Is There a Teen Suicide Crisis?: Or are Social Scientists After More Federal Research Funds?, WASH. POST, Jan. 25, 1987 at B5, col. 1.

See, Del Bello, Needed: A U.S. Commission on Teen-Age Suicide, N.Y. TIMES, Sept. 12, 1984, at A31, col. 1.

See also, Gelman & Gangelhoff, Teen-age Suicide in the Sun Belt, NEWSWEEK, Aug. 15, 1983, at 70, where it is stated that every year approximately 5,000 teenagers kill themselves and as many as half a million more make attempts, that in turn conduces to a 300 percent increase in adolescent suicides since 1955.

128. Id.

129. Carlson, supra note 127.

130. McCormack, High-Achieving Teen-Agers Tell of Considering Suicide, WASH. POST, Sept. 14, 1986, at A7, col. 1.

131. Id.

132. Id.

See Peck, Towards a Theory of Suicide: The Case for Modern Fatalism, 11 OMEGA 1 (1990-81).

133. Streitfield, The Aftermath of Suicides: Attention Must be Paid, but How Much and at What Price?, WASH. POST, May 25, 1987, at C5, col. 1.

See also, Dobbs, Four N.J. Teenagers Commit Suicide, WASH. POST, Mar. 12, 1987, at A3, col. 3; 2 Illinois Suicides Similar to New Jersey Teen-Agers, WASH. POST, Mar. 14, 1987, at A3, col. 1.

134. Russell, Teen-Age Suicides Linked to TV Coverage of Subject, WASH. POST, Sept. 11, 1986, at A3, col. 5.

135. Id.

See also, Phillips & Carstensen, Clustering of Teenage Suicides After Television Stories about Suicide, 315 NEW ENG. J. MED. 685 (Sept. 11, 1986).

136. Streitfield, supra note 133.

137. Id.

138. Id.

139. Price, Pro Suicide Activists Call for Right to Assist. WASH. TIMES, Mar. 13, 1987, at 6A, col. 2 (quoting Prof. Margaret P. Battin, Univ. of Utah at Salt Lake City).

140. Farberow, Indirect Self-Destructive Behavior: Classification and Characteristics in THE MANY FACES OF SUICIDE 15, 19 (N. Faberow ed. 1980).

Other destructive behaviors are listed as: mountain climbing; scuba diving; hand gliding; trapeze performs in circuses; stuntmen; boat racing and violent contact sports (boxing). Id.

141. Id. at 17.

142. Litman, Psychodynamics of Indirect Self-Destructive Behavior in THE MANY FACES OF SUICIDE 28 (N. Faberow ed. 1980).

143. Id. at 39.

144. Id.

145. Id.

146. Achte, The Psychopathology of Indirect Self-Destruction in THE MANY FACES OF SUICIDE 41 (N. Faberow ed. 1980).

147. Id. at 51.

148. Delk, High-Risk Sports as Indirect Self-Destructive Behavior in THE MANY FACES OF SUICIDE 393 at 395 (N. Faberow ed. 1980).

149. Id.

150. D. de Cantanzo, SUICIDE AND SELF–DAMAGING BEHAVIOR 21 (1981).

See L. TRIBE, AMERICAN CONSTITUTIONAL LAW 938 *passim* (1978) for an analysis of governmental interference with life styles—recreational (motorcycling) and otherwise.

151. Supra note 148 at 406.

152. Id.

153. Id.

154. Duncan, Public Policy and the AIDS Epidemic, 2 J. CONTEMP. HEALTH L. & POL'Y 169 (1986).

155. TIME, July 7, 1980 at 49.

156. Subsequent page references are to the pamphlet.

157. A GUIDE TO SELF–DELIVERANCE 1 (1981).

158. Id. at 16–23.

159. Id. at 9.

160. Id. at 10.

161. Id.

162. Id. at 15.

163. Id. at 4.

164. Id. at 6.

165. Id. at 4.

166. R. v. Nicholas Reed, [1982] Crim. L. R. 819.

167. Id.

168. Id.

169. Attorney General v. Able and others, [1984] 1 All E.R. 277.

170. Id.

171. Id. at 288.

172. Id.

173. 9 & 10 Eliz. II c. 60 (1961).

174. See G. WILLIAMS, TEXTBOOK OF CRIMINAL LAW 578 (1983).

175. Id.

176. Id.

177. Id. at 579.

178. Id.

179. Id. Maubouche, Final Choices: Popular Suicide Guide Enrages the French, WASH. POST, Sept. 6, 1982, at C1, col. 6.

180. Id.

181. Id.

182. Rational Suicide Raises Patient Rights Issues, 66 A.B.A.J. 1499 (1980).

183. TIME Mag., Mar. 21, 1985 at 85.

184. Supra note 217.

185. *Martin v. Struthers*, 319 U.S. 141, 143 (1943).

186. J. ROBERTSON, THE RIGHTS OF THE CRITICALLY ILL 30 (1983).
    See generally, J. NOWAK, R. ROTUNDA, J. YOUNG, CONSTITUTIONAL LAW, Ch. 18 (2d ed. 1983).

187. See e.g., *Heffron v. Int'l Soc. for Krishna Consciousness, Inc.* 452 U.S. 640 (1981).

188. Supra notes 64–76.
    See also, ROBERTSON, supra note 186 at 29, 30.

189. Supra note 186.

190. Supra note 183.

191. Branderburg v. State of Ohio, 395 U.S. 44, 23 L. Ed. 2d 420 (1969).

192. _____ U.S. _____, 23 L. Ed. 2d at 439.

193. Id.

194. Survey, Euthanasia: Criminal, Tort, Constitutional and Legislative Considerations, 48 NOTRE DAME L. REV. 1202, 1206 (1973).

195. A similar "moral" problem exists with the free distribution, without prosecution, of terrorist manuals that describe how bridges may be blown up and human lives thus brought into chaos. G. WILLIAMS, TEXTBOOK OF CRIMINAL LAW 340, at n. 11 (1983).

196. See supra notes 64–76.

In Texas, as early as 1902, it was determined that since suicide was not illegal, it could not be held to be a crime to aid a criminal act. *Grace v. State,* 44 TEX. CRIM. 193, 194, 69 S.W. 529, 530 (1902).

In 1908, it was held suicide assistance must be passive—not active—to be a defense to murder. Accordingly, to shoot an individual upon request would equate with active suicide for which the acting party would be charged with murder in the first degree. *Sanders v. State,* 54 Tex. Crim. 101, 105 112 S.W. 68, 70 (1908).

And, in New Jersey, in 1901, in *Campbell v. Supreme Conclave, Improved Order of Heptasophs,* it was held that since suicide was not a crime, the public good would not prevent one from taking his life that "may be worthless to the public." 66 N.J. 274, 49 A. 550, 553 (1901). *But see, State v. Ehlers,* 98 N.J.L. 236, 238. 119 A. 15 (1922) where punishment was given for an attempted suicide.

197. Comment, The Right to Die, 7 HOUS. L. REV. 654, 656 (1970). In *State v. Cobb,* 229 Kan. 522, 625 P. 2d 1133 (1981) the state supreme court sustained a conviction for a charge of first degree murder of the defendant who—acting upon the decedent's request—injected him with an overdose of cocaine and then proceeded to shoot him.

In 1986, Roswell Gilbert, 75, was sentenced to life imprisonment for the premeditated murder of his 51 year old wife. He shot her twice in the head thereby seeking to end her painful and progressively degenerative conditions of osteoporosis and Alzeheimer's disease. Gilbert v. State, 487 So. 2d 1185 (Fla. 1986).

In Australia, aiding and abetting the death of another by his own hand is a crime punished as a homocide. Sharma, Euthanasia in Australasia, 2 J. CONTEMP. HEALTH L. & POL'Y 131, 139 (1986).

See generally, Shaffer, Criminal Liability for Assisting Suicide, 86 COLUM. L. REV. 348 (1986).

198. Survey, Euthanasia: Criminal, Tort, Constitutional and Legislative Considerations, 48 NOTRE DAME L. REV. 1202, 1206 (1973).

See Vesey, She Wanted to Die, So He Killed Her: Man Gets Probation as Dead Woman's Family Praises His Devotion, WASH. POST, NOV. 24, 1985, at 1, col. 1 (story of a Maryland woman who decided to kill herself, gave a gun to her friend and asked him to pull the trigger).

199. See Anno., 95 A.L.R. 2d 175, 191 *passim* (1964) (person other than actor liable

for manslaughter); ARIZ. REV. STAT. ANN. 13-1103 (1978); COLO. REV. STAT. 18-3-104 (1978); CONN. GEN. STAT. 53a-56 (1981); ORE. REV. STAT. 163.125 (1981).

See also, *Regina v. Creamer,* Ct. of Criminal Appeal [1965] 3 All E. R. 257, where it was determined, "A man is guilty of involuntary manslaughter when he intends an unlawful act and one likely to do harm to the person and death results which was neither foreseen nor intended. It is the accident of death resulting which makes him guilty of manslaughter as opposed to some lesser offense, such as assault. . . . "

200. See e.g., *Stephenson v. State,* 205 Ind. 141, 179 N.E. (1932) where shame and disgrace lead to a (coerced) suicide so as to amount to a killing by him who inflicted it. Here, after the decedent was subject to two days of various sexual perversions, she bought six tablets of bichloride of mercury and ingested them in an effort to commit suicide. She was initially unsuccessful in this act, but ten days later she died— apparently of a combination of shock, loss of food and rest, a reaction to the poison and infection and lack of proper treatment.

201. See e.g., J. HALL, GENERAL PRINCIPLES OF CRIMINAL LAW 115, 123, 131–33 (2d ed. 1960).

Recklessness charges may arise even though the actor believed harm would not occur or is indifferent whether or not it occurs or, traditionally, is grossly ignorant or criminally inattentive to his actions. Id. 115, 123.

202. Hall, supra, at 114, 116, 120, 127.

203. The Model Penal Code, §2.03(b) (Proposed Official Draft, 1963).

204. Id. at §2.03(3).

205. Model Penal Code (Tent. Draft No. 4, Comments §2.03 at 133–134 (1955).

206. 66 A.B.A.J. 1499, 1501 (1980).

207. Id.

208. Id.

209. Id.

210. Id.

211. Id.

Over the last twenty-five years or so, both suicide and attempted suicide have lost the status of crimes. G. GRIEZ, J.M. BOYLE, JR., LIFE AND DEATH WITH LIBERTY AND JUSTICE 122 (1979).

212. Rational Suicide Raises Patient Rights Issue, 66 A.B.A.J. 1499, 1501 (1980).

213. Id.

See also, Appelbaum & Roth, Patients Who Refuse Treatment in Medical Hospitals, 250 J.A.M.A. 1296 (1983).

214. Engelhardt & Malloy, Suicide and Assisting Suicide: A Critique of Legal Sanctions, 36 SO. W. L. J. 1003, 1021 (1982).

Interestingly, the Supreme Court of Georgia ruled that based upon the consti- tutional right of privacy (and placing reliance on denial of medical treatment cases) a prisoner could starve himself to death and the state had no right to destroy such a person's will by frustrating his attempt to die in order to make a point or make a statement. *Zant v. Prevante,* 248 Ga. 832, 834, 286 S.E. 2d 715, 717 (1982).

215. Id. at 1037.

It has been argued that although attempted suicide should be recognized as a crime, it should not always be treated as such. Rather, the courts should assert a power to drop the criminal charge and require the defendant to undergo psychiatric and medical treatment. C. RICE, THE VANISHING RIGHT TO LIVE 81 (1969).

216. Id.

217. Id.

218. See generally, Williams, The Right to Die, 134 NEW L.J. 73 (Jan. 27, 1984); Williams, The Right to Commit Suicide in MORAL PROBLEMS IN MEDICINE at 388 (S. GOROWITZ et al eds. 1976). Professor Williams observes, "It is still not fully recognized that everyone has not merely a legal but a moral right to drink the hemlock, so far as society in general is concerned." Id. at 388.

219. Ringel, Suicide Prevention and The Value of Human Life in SUICIDE: THE PHILOSOPHICAL ISSUES at 206 (M. BATTIN, D. MAYO eds. 1980).

220. Id.

221. Id. at 207, 208.

222. Id. at 209.

223. Id. at 210.

See Shneidman & Faberow, The Suicide Prevention Center of Los Angeles in SUICIDAL BEHAVIORS: DIAGNOSIS AND MANAGEMENT at 367 (H. RESNIK ed. 1968).

224. Id.

225. Id.

226. Fox, The Samaritans in SUICIDAL BEHAVIORS: DIAGNOSIS AND MANAGEMENT at 405 (H. RESNIK ed. 1968).

227. Id.

228. Id.

229. Id.

230. Id.

231. Id. at 406.

232. Fox, The Recent Decline of Suicide in Britain: The Role of the Samaritan Suicide Prevention Movement in SUICIDOLOGY: CONTEMPORARY DEVELOPMENTS at 504, 512 *passim* (E. SHNEIDMAN ed. 1976).

See generally Stengel, Lay Organizations and Suicide Prevention in THE SAMARITANS at 107 (C. VARAH ed. 1965).

233. Brandt, The Morality and Rationality of Suicide in SUICIDOLOGY: CONTEMPORARY DEVELOPMENTS at 397, 399 (E. SHNEIDMAN ed. 1976).

234. Farberow & Shneidman, A Survey of Agencies for The Prevention of Suicide in THE CRY FOR HELP at 136, 137 (N. FARBEROW, E. SHNEIDMAN eds. 1961).

235. Id.

236. Id.

237. J. MEERLOO, SUICIDE AND MASS SUICIDE 174 (1968).

See generally, P. MANDELKORN, HOW TO PREVENT SUICIDE (1967).

238. Id.

239. Id.

240. Supra note 234 at 6.

241. Id.

See Schulman, Suicide and Suicide Prevention: A Legal Analysis, 54 A.B.A.J. 855, 860–862 (1968).

242. The Volunteer Suicidologist: Current Status and Future Prospects in SUI-CIDOLOGY: CONTEMPORARY DEVELOPMENTS at 480, 481 (E. SHNEIDMAN ed. 1961).

243. Id.

244. Id.

245. Greenberg, Involuntary Psychiatric Commitments to Prevent Suicide, 49 N.Y. Univ. L. Rev. 227 (1974).

When, in 1972, New Jersey abolished the criminal offense of attempted suicide, it provided for the involuntary commitment for those attempting unsuccessfully the act. See N.J. STAT. ANN. 2C:11-6, 2C:3-7(e); 30:4-26:3 (West 1982).

246. Greenberg, supra at 229.

247. Id.

248. Id.

249. Greensburg, supra note 245 at 233.

250. Id. at 334.

251. Id.

252. Id. at 232.

253. Id.

254. Id.

255. D. de Cantanzo, SUICIDE AND SELF DAMAGING BEHAVIOUR, Ch. 11 (1984).

256. Id. at 142.

257. Id.

258. Greensberg, supra note 245 at 223.

259. Id.

260. Id.

See Kjervik, The Psychotherapist's Duty to Act Reasonably to Prevent Suicide: A Proposal to Allow Rational Suicide, 2 BEHAVIORIAL SCIENCES & THE LAW 207 (1984).

261. LaFond, The Empirical Consequences and Policy Implications of Broadening the Statutory Criteria for Civil Commitment, 3 YALE L. & POL'Y REV. 395 (1985); Morse, A Preference for Liberty: The Case Against Involuntary Commitment of the Mentally Disordered, 70 CAL. L. REV. 54 (1982).

262. Herman, Barriers to Providing Effective Treatment: A Critique of Revision in Procedural, Substantive, and Dispositional Criteria in Involuntary Civil Commitment, 39 VAND. L. REV. 84, 85 (1986).

263. Id. at 89.

264. Id. at 92.

265. Id. at 86.

266. Id.

267. Rhoden, The Limits of Liberty: Deinstitutionalization, Homelessness and Libertarian Theory, 31 EMORY L. J. 375 (1982).

268. In 1955, there were 559,000 patients in mental hospitals; in 1980, approxi-

mately 138,000. GOLDMAN, ADAMS & TAUBE, DEINSTITUTIONALIZATION: THE DATA DEMYTHOLOGIZED 129, 131 (1983).

269. See, THE LEAST RESTRICTIVE ALTERNATIVES: PRINCIPLES & PRACTICES (H. TURNBULL ed. 1981).

270. Myers, Involuntary Civil Commitment of The Mentally Ill: A System in Need of Change, 29 VILL. L. REV. 367, 414 (1983-84).

271. Szasz, On the Legitimacy of Psychiatric Power, 14 RUTGERS L. REV. 479 (1983).

272. Supra note 270 at 412.

273. Id.

It has been suggested that an ideal suicide prevention policy would: "save through methods entailing minimal unpleasantness, the lives of as many as possible of those who do not wish to die; interfere as little as possible with those who after some change of consideration persist in wanting to die and afford maximum protection against interference with the liberty of those who pose no threat of suicide." See Greenberg, supra note 245 at 242, 243.

274. Herman, Barriers to Providing Effective Treatment: A Critique of Revision in Procedural, Substantive, and Dispositional Criteria in Involuntary Civil Commitment, 39 VAND. L. REV. 84, 94 (1986).

See also, S. BRAKEL, J. PARRY & B. WEINER, THE MENTALLY DISABLED AND THE LAW 33-37 (2d ed. 1985).

275. Id. at 95.

276. Id.

277. Id. at 96.

278. Id. at 100.

See generally, Goleman, States Move to Ease Law Committing Mentally Ill: Greater Readiness to Hospitalize Marks Shift in Battle over Patients Rights, N.Y. TIMES, Dec. 9, 1986 at Y19, col. 1.

279. BRAKEL, PARRY & WEINER, supra note 274 at 37.

280. Dresser, Bound to Treatment: The Ulysses Contract, HASTINGS CENTER RPT. 13 (June 1984).

281. Id.

282. Id.

283. Id. at 15.

284. Id.

285. Id.

286. Id.

See also, J. CHILDRESS, LIBERTY, PATERNALISM & HEALTH CARE 69 (1979).

287. See Stromberg & Stone, A Model State Law on Civil Commitment of The Mentally Ill, 20 HARV. J. LEGIS. 275 (1983).

288. Id. at 321 (Sec. 4).

289. Id. at 330.

290. Id. at 331.

291. Id. at 335.

292. Id.

See generally, Note, The Role of Law in Suicide Prevention: Beyond Civil Commitment — A Bystander Duty to Report Suicide Threats, 39 STAN. L. REV. 929 (1987).

Chapter II

THE PHILOSOPHICAL PERSPECTIVE

Even though philosophical arguments and issues are rarely isolated within well-defined context and thus give rise to widely disbursed and disturbing repercussions,[1] any medico-legal exegesis of suicide, euthanasia and self-determination must tackle the undergriding ethical, moral and philosophical tenets of the subject area and thereby structure a framework for principle analysis and a construct for decision making.

Today, life—and the maintenance of physical life—has become a common and, indeed, intense preoccupation; one based upon an assumption of the unnatural nature of death and the need to arrest or delay it at any cost, no matter the brevity of the opportunity.[2] Instead of seeking, realizing and thereupon maintaining an ideal of human rationality whereby mature and rational individuals not only live with but accept and incorporate into their specific life plans the realities of human existence and of human mortality,[3] death has become a manifestation of demonic power to be mastered and overcome by advanced medical technologies.[4]

> Dramatic medical interventions portrayed in the media become living "westerns." The powers of death are the bad guys, to be vanquished by the good guys, dressed in white coats, rather than white hats. Every delay of death is a victory by the forces of good.[5]

While it has been suggested that behind the ordering of all normal functioning is the fear of death and that, consequently, self-preservation is a primary goal, an ever-present fear of this type could be totally debilitating. Thus, in order to allow for any form of normal living to take place, the fear must be repressed and with this comes an approaching understanding of the paradox of recognizing an ever-present fear of death as a normal process of biological functioning, an instinct for self-preservation yet—in conscious life—a presumed obliviousness to this very fear.[6] "Man, may in fact, be thought of as lying to himself, about himself and about his world"—with this fear of knowledge of himself being a major cause of many psychological illnesses.[7] Yet, in the world of reality, everyone should realize that this fight with death is a battle which is truly lost before it ever commences; for death *is* the ultimate reality. The outcome of the battle is not the reward. But, the uniqueness of the confrontation and its hoped-for beauty is to be found in the dignity of the actual struggle and the manner in which the end is recorded.[8]

A SENSE OF PROFANATION: A TWO-EDGED SWORD

While it is proper to consider a person's life as sacrosanct and to exhibit an attitude of awe, reverence and support toward it, with an ending of it as a "profanation of the sacred," is it not as much a profanation to witness an individual whose life is prolonged at an agonizing level of pain and indignity?[9]

> Not being able to choose death when death is experienced as an essential benefit, could easily seem degrading and profaning of personhood. Why should the disease have all the say, and the patient none? By succumbing to such moral determinism, is not the sacred power of deliberation and choice profaned?[10]

For better or worse, depending upon one's set of values, respect for life and its inherent value is being considered more and more an inextricable function of the quality of life.[11] Indeed, a fundamental issue in this present exegesis is whether attitudes and principles of quality of life *are* to be adjudged or more value and significance than life *qua* life. Life is a sacred value, to be sure. But is the value of human life a single and isolated value? Its determinative significance is best tested and achieved when it is compared with other values. "Without life other things are of no value to us, but by the same token without other things life may be of no value to us."[12]

If the binding force of life is to be recognized as love, a proper argument can be made that advocates efforts be undertaken to maximize responses to love in all life situations. Thus, if an act that is undertaken would bestow a greater degree of harm than good not only to the concerned individual but to those around him, it should not be completed. In order to maintain a resolution of the conundrum here, the crucial point to be understood is that a cost/benefit analysis is inevitably performed—either consciously or unconsciously—and that love should be the basic normative value used in each situation to resolve the balancing test.[13] While recognizing the inherent worth of the individual, situations will develop in which no cognizable benefits are realizable from a prolongation of physical existence. And, as such, to maintain "life" would be regarded as an indignity.[14] Indeed, the Roman Catholic Church has never insisted of the physician that he use every available means in order to sustain human life; only that he not undertake positive acts that are calculated to end a patient's life.[15]

It is increasingly difficult to justify—from a moral viewpoint—letting one be given over to a pitilessly slow and dehumanizing death than it is to justify assisting him to escape that misery in the most beneficial and humane manner.[16] One of the foremost moral philosophers of the day, Richard A. McCormick, has stated legal concepts of privacy and the common law right of self-determination are inadequate bases for moral justifications by competent patients regarding the appropriateness of acceptance or refusal of medical treatment.[17] Rather, a more comprehensive moral base for justification of treatment refusal is either the burdensomeness of the treatment, itself, or its uselessness.[18]

For the incompetent individual or one who, while competent, never expressed himself on the issue of emergency care and treatment, two additional mechanisms may be utilized in actual cases of extremity: the principle of patient benefit, with the determination of the patient's best interests being made by the family—consistent with the principle of familial autonomy or self-determination.[19] Accordingly, the state should only intervene in non-treatment decisions "when the familial judgment so exceeds the limits of reason that the compromise with what is objectively in the incompetent's best interests cannot be tolerated."[20]

MORAL PHILOSOPHY

When entering the field of moral philosophy, it must be remembered, "that no action is instrinsically right or wrong, nothing is inherently good or evil."[21] Experiments of rightness or wrongness are but ethical terms.[22] "Values and the morality of human acts are contingent, depending on the shape of the action in the situation."[23] Accordingly, the variables and the factors found within each particular set of circumstances are, in truth, "the determinants of what ought to be done."[24] Logic neither allows proof nor defense of values, rather, they are established by an admixture of choice, conditioning and commitment.[25]

Invariably, human "rights" are blended and, thus, confused with right conduct. Humanistic ethics hold that when an act "helps" human beings, it is classified as a right. What confers the propriety of action here is, simply, human need.[26] If human rights are recognized as not self-validating nor intrinsically valid in and of themselves, the question must be raised as to the manner by which they are validated.[27] "It is need that validates rights, not the other way around."[28] Thus, when an act of suicide helps an individual in the fulfillment of a need, call it self-determination, autonomy or self-deliverance, it is a right choice.[29]

Another philosophical view would hold that being recognized as "at liberty" to undertake an act should not be recognized further as bestowing the status of a fundamental right upon that liberty.[30] Thus, a person seeking to commit suicide or in fact committing the act should not properly be considered as asserting a self-defeating claim to a right of destruction of any rights which he might possess—but rather only a claim to abridge or destroy a liberty: here, a liberty to bring an end to life.[31] In a word, "Suicide is the signature of freedom."[32] Or, considered otherwise, the act of suicide is but an assertion of the right of autonomy or self-determination. Viewed thusly, then, this liberty to kill oneself would impose upon all other members of society a duty not to interfere with another's act of suicide. It would be just as much a violation of an individual's autonomy to deter him from carrying out such an act as it would be a violation of his same rights of self-determination to impose non-consensual medical care upon him. Accordingly, if there are no issues regarding competency in focus, it could be argued that it would be morally impermissible for one to interfere with a decision by a competent terminally ill individual to take his own life. Of course, no moral obligation (unless perhaps one arising from a consent killing, death pact[33] or perceived family obligation) would exist and thus impose a responsibility for another to either facilitate or give primary assistance to one wishing suicide.

If liberty to kill oneself were to be recognized as guaranteed by some aspect of the right of privacy or as a fundamental right comparable to that of speech and religion, it would be subject to control or being overriden by a compelling state interest.[34] The preferred analysis for the moral philosopher is to maintain that the liberty to kill oneself is little more "than immunity from criminal prosecution and from such interference as would have no rational relationship to any legitimate state interest."[35] Yet, since the states concern with preserving life has been recognized and fostered as a fundamental interest or concern (surely, a rational one at that) from the early days of its power of *parens patriae,* this preferred analysis will be difficult to sustain.[36] There are slow, but perceptible judicial indications and legislative directions, however, that give rise to a belief that enlightened self-determination both for the terminally ill competent as well as the protected incompetent is gaining in acceptability and that the states obsessive concern with life *qua* life is being conditioned by *quality* of life standards.[37]

More and more, the controlling ethical question no longer emerges as to how death is defined but, rather, who controls or manages—in its formal sense—the manner and the timing of death. Stated otherwise, the pivotal question is who possesses the right to decide when treatment should be terminated or when heroic or extraordinary measures should be undertaken.[38]

If it is assumed as a given right that man seeks, through his living, to achieve a good or virtuous (i.e., moral) life, it should follow that he should be provided with supporting "ideal rights" or those means available to achieve the good life.[39] The fundamental requisites of a good (moral) life, then, are to be found in the ideal rights to life, itself, and to death.[40] If this latter or co-ordinate ideal right to die is construed accordingly "as the right to determine the manner and timing of one's own death,"[41] it would form an inextricable part of the good life,

> for dying should be something that relates a person intimately to others as a moral agent and that is closely bound up with his personal moral values and ideals. . . . Society should recognize the ideal right to die a good death, a death that is not simply a painless and dignified death, but one that could have moral quality.[42]

Societal recognition of an ideal right to die forces upon it an obligation to not only permit, but facilitate, individual control over death and the dying process. This recognition can be achieved legally through application and enforcement of the laws of privacy.[43]

In the final analysis, the controlling issue should not be tied to a rights issue as much as to a question regarding the ultimate task of medicine.[44] It is a reasonable, just and humane goal of medicine—a non-delegable duty of all physicians—to keep a "naturally doomed body" from expiring? Should a captive patient, because of his physical impotence, have his right of self-determination disenfranchised by health care providers?[45] Should not the patient in an irreversible coma expect those attending to his care to have a recognized or co-ordinate duty to terminate his care by a withdrawal of life support systems.[46] Simply put, the true goal of

medicine and the duty of its physicians who serve it should be to make
dying more gentle and humane, less violent in its nature and certainly
not an extended economic catastrophe.[47]

AUTONOMY

Because of the various meanings and subtleties of autonomy that defy
definitive agreement, it is better to study the social uses of it as a
principle in order to thereby approach an understanding of its use and
application as the center most force in the present analysis.

If it is accepted as a given right that autonomy is a shared or reciprocal
principle—and one that is "the controlling fulcrum in the obligations"
one may owe to others, and they to him, a vexatious conundrum is presented.[48] If recognition of autonomy is a mutually shared principle, how
may a moral obligation thought to exist between and among individuals
be either met or extinguished by a unilateral declaration of autonomy?[49]
Thus, if a patient expresses his wish to die to the attending physician, is
the physician's belief, felt-duty or "obligation" to save that particular life,
overridden by such declaration? As understood in the common autonomy doctrine, the patient's expression or choice of his own moral good
would preclude others from assuming or asserting those on behalf of the
patient.[50]

The principal dilemma, then, is to decide whether—upon a patient's
declaration or assertion of autonomy or enlightened self-determination—
a physician's moral obligation vanishes or is but overridden by a high
fundamental value? "The moral autonomy of others does not rule out
non—coercive attempts to persuade them to think or act differently."[51]
What cannot be done is to *impose* a distinct and contrary values or
the dictates of another's conscience upon them in a non-voluntary manner.
This, then, is the crucial determining point regarding moral autonomy:
personal liberty allows a restriction of actions asserted or taken by others
against or on behalf of an individual.[52] "Only a voluntary ceding of
suspension of autonomy rights can change the nature of that relationship
with others."[53] An acceptance of autonomy's use and application is an
obvious hazard to the working concept of both moral relationships and
moral community. Yet, it is acknowledged from time to time that justice
(often under the guise of paternalism) allows individual liberties to
be suppressed.[54]

The dignity, power and correctness of John Stuart Mills's words written in 1859 in his essay, "On Liberty," should be as much a part of our thinking in this area of analysis and as significant now as they were in his social setting in England when they were first penned. Asserting the object of the essay to be the articulation of a very basic principle—"that the sole end for which mankind are warranted individually, or collectively, in interfering with the liberty of action of any of their number, is self-protection," Mill continues by stating,

> .... That the only purpose for which power can be rightfully exercised over any member of a civilized community, against his will, is to prevent harm to others. His own good, either physical or moral, is not a sufficient warrant.[55]

His closing observation is that the individual should be recognized as "sovereign" over his "own body and mind."[56]

The free choices made by autonomous human beings must always be respected. Here, the operative concept is autonomous, which should be equated with competent. The revitalization and emphasis placed upon the concept of autonomy emerged during the 1970's as a response to medical and social (state) paternalism that had grown in power and scope of application for centuries.[57] Indeed, one distinguished authority has expressed his impression that, "autonomy has supplanted eudomonia (happiness), or utility, or the glorification of God as the good to be maximized by ethical behavior."[58]

Although suicide may appear to exemplify autonomy at its highest level of explication, and affect only one person, a closer examination reveals the fact that the person attempting suicide is also a citizen, a member of a family or other organization and perhaps even a patient. Thus, the state, his family members, contractual or business partners and various physicians and health care providers may well have an interest in his life and a concern for his actions. Even if the person contemplating a suicide is determined at one particular time to undertake it, events may change and various therapies employed that bring a total change in initial perspective.

Autonomy, or as modern courts choose to denominate it, "privacy," is seen as being promoted as the central value in contemporary medical practice.[59] As more and more courts begin to recognize and develop autonomy as an inherent right to die with whatever level of dignity that may exist under the particular circumstances, the right to live—it has been suggested—is de-emphasized.[60] Traditionally, autonomy of patient choice was never held in high regard by the medical profession—for, it was always maintained that the health care providers were more uniquely qualified to determine the court of treatment for patients than the patients themselves.[61] Interestingly, qualitative life was, instinctively, the measuring rod for medical action or inaction—as the case might warrant.[62] With a widening judicial recognition of privacy rights, which of necessity forces consideration of qualitative living, the courts appear to be re-affirming what has been accepted medical practice for years; but only under a different principle or standard.[63] *Just* results are the judicial goals and extending suffering from a terminal illness or death, itself, is simply not just.

It has been suggested, further, that the quality of life issue is reduceable to a simple question of whether a patient's life is worth *saving*.[64] Caution has been urged here because—it is postured—that once health "is reduced to one value among many, and death is often seen as preferable to life," physicians and health care providers find it less complicated to simply "let people refuse care than to struggle with them."[65] Indeed, when law casts confusing shadows in this area of concern, physicians begin to think first and foremost of minimizing their own risks and "often call in their lawyers and do what they are told" acting as though they were but common bureaucrats.[66]

While the central importance of patient autonomy in the medical decision making process is an acknowledged given, as a legally recognizable and protectable interest, it has yet to be recognized.[67] Indeed, it has only been elevated to a level of concern because of the interplay of two other complementary interests: that of bodily security, protected as such by legal rules against unconsented contact and bodily well-being, that is, in turn, protected by canons that structure and maintain professional competence.[68] Yet, neither of these interests can stand rightly as a substitute for a legal protectable and recognizable right of autonomy or self-determination.[69]

Traditionally, because of their medical knowledge and the hierarchical role society has conferred upon them, physicians have often acted out of normal course in pre-empting patient authority in medical decision making.[70] The very selection of a physician by a patient was seen as a complete delegation of all authority by the patient to participate in his subsequent medical treatment.[71] Recently, however, over the past several decades, with phenomenal advances in medical technology have come numerous options for patient care. This level of increased knowledge has been fed to society by the popular press and television media provoking much debate and public comment.[72] It is now becoming more and more apparent that those persons about whom decisions are made regarding their medical needs both wish and demand to be involved directly in the decision making process.[73] Thus, today, a shift from professional dominance toward individual knowledge and self-determination is being seen.[74] The law has not responded however in a forceful and directive manner to recognize patient autonomy.[75]

Since a physician's authority derives solely from the patient, it should extend or contract as the competent patient directs.[76] As a matter of professional competence, the physician should have a duty to disclose, whatever materially relevant information and possibilities which he possesses, to his patient so that the patient may be—in turn—enabled to decide what course of medical treatment (or non-treatment) is to be followed.[77]

Medical decisions affecting the level of health care to be provided a patient "depend upon moral values, economic considerations and risk preference, as well as on medical expertise."[78] Since these decisions "affect the patient more directly than anyone else, the patient's choices, education but not pre-empted by the doctor's expertise, should be controlling."[79] Patient autonomy should, indeed, be recognized as well as protected to the same degree as any other distinct legal interest;[80] for what an individual is and wants to do with his life are among the most basic expressions of self-determination.[81]

PATERNALISM

Paternalism may be defined classically as, "a refusal to accept or to acquiesce in another person's wishes, choices and actions for that person's own benefits."[82] Thus, the two primary underpinnings of paternalism are recognized as altruistic beneficence (where the purpose is to act in order to confer a benefit upon another) and a rejection of the wishes, choices or actions of another under certain circumstances.[83] The principle of beneficence is forever being asserted as either a justification for or a defense of paternalism.[84]

In order to justify exercises of medical paternalism or paternalistic intervention, an "at risk" medical situation must be recognized where a high probability of harm would result to the person *in extremis* unless a course of intervention were followed.[85] Secondly, under usual circumstances where a decision has been made by an individual regarding health care, no questions regarding the competence of that patient will be made unless the decision, itself, appears to be mistaken; that is, the patient did not understand or deliberate rationally in reaching the questioned decision.[86] The third and final condition that must be met in order to justify an exercise of medical paternalism is that the probable benefit of a positive intervention should outweigh the probable harm of inaction or, here, non-intervention.[87] Termed, proportionality, what is sought is a validation or proof that the benefit accruing from the intervention will not only outweigh those moral rules that make some actions (as, for example, lying and coercion) in and of themselves wrong, but also any goods or positive values a patient will severely jeopardize or lose through such paternalistic actions.[88]

Obviously, a physician's own personal values shape—to a great extent—the nature and degree to which he will exhibit paternalism in his relations with his patients.[89] Altruism, however, does not alone guide this sense or spirit of paternalism; for the values to which a physician subscribes are also not only by self-interest and by professional bias, but by personal needs—any or all of which may be in conflict with the patient's best interests.[90] Research agendas, professional training opportunities and personal ethical views all combine to create a professional bias of one degree or other in medical decision making for the critically ill.[91] Accordingly, in order to stave off personal sense of failure or defeat, some physicians view death as the real and only enemy of professional medicine and muster all aggressive efforts within their power to fight and "win" (no matter, momentarily) the battle. Humane and compassionate care for the suffering is supplanted by what is considered "machine medicine."[92] Other physicians utilize new technologies as a substitute for their practical inexperience; and still others will choose a course of aggressive treatment because the particular at-risk patient presents, with his own case, an opportunity for the physician to better develop his skills.[93] "Doctors with state-of-the-art skills want to use them, and may derive aesthetic satisfaction when they do."[94] Thus it can be seen that vigilance must ever be maintained in order to safeguard against the physicians' ready eagerness to substitute one form or other "motivated" paternalism for his patient's right of enlightened self-determination.

TELEOLOGICAL AND DEONTOLOGICAL
ARGUMENTS REGARDING SUICIDE

In essence, there are two sets of arguments propounded when any critical analysis of suicide is undertaken: the teleological and the deontological. The teleological arguments—or arguments *against* suicide— are grounded in a simple syllogism:

1. Actions that tend to maximize good are right and those that tend to evil are wrong.
2. Suicide is an action that tends to maximize evil.
3. Therefore, suicide is wrong.[95]

It is readily seen that while each of the three arguments assert suicide tends to maximize evil and is thus wrong, they differ not only in the definition of evil but in the scope of the consequences considered therefrom. Each of the arguments also differ regarding what good or goods are the more decisive.[96] In order to determine the significance of the goods, they must be weighed or balanced according to a hierarchical value system that measures their significance in each case under consideration.[97]

The central teleological argument is that suicide is an act resulting in external damnation.[98] To sustain the intellectual validity of this supposition another syllogism is structured which asserts:

1. The deity is displeased by heinous acts that result in eternal damnation.
2. Without question, suicide is a heinous act.
3. Therefore, the deity is displeased by such acts of suicide that result in eternal damnation.[99]

The fatal flaw in this argument is that there is no verifiable evidence that suicide is either damnable or displeasing to the deity.[100] Since neither the Old nor the New Testament explicity condemn suicide,[101] for it to be taken as a heinous act sbustantiation of this fact must derive from the Sixth Commandment—"Thou shalt not kill." Yet, by way of reply, one could assert simply that it is quite an arbitrary posture to assume, without more, that this was the full import of this Commandment.[102]

A second and far more compelling argument against suicide is presented when it is asserted that the act, itself, is harmful to both family and friends.[103] If familial and collegial relations are so significant to the efficacy of this argument, if one had neither family nor friends, the act would be without criticism.[104] If negative consequences flowing from an act of suicide to family and friends are the pivotal issues of the act's rightness or wrongness, "suicide would be right (and possibly even mandatory) if it would benefit one's family and friends rather than burden them!"[105] A balancing mechanism might well have to be employed that would attempt to weigh the pain caused both the family and the friends of the suicide against the possible benefits to them as well as the possible benefits accruing to others and to the society at large.[106]

Suppose, for example, that an individual is suffering with an incurable disease and that the costs of his maintenance are considerable. While his family may not want him to die and his suicide might well cause them considerable pain and anguish, his suicide could also benefit other hospital patients needing the hospital resources allocated currently to his care. An argument could thus be made that in order to decide whether an act of suicide maximizes evil or—contrariwise—maximizes good, the consequences to a wider range of persons and a wider range of goods must be considered. Accordingly, it is submitted that where an act of suicide produces more good than evil for the whole of society, it would be right and proper and not wrong.[107]

The "argument from precedent" accepts premises only two and four of the "wedge" argument or in other words that, "Action A is similar to action B in morally relevant ways," and "To do A is therefore to establish a precedent for (or remove a precedent against) B" thus "Action B is undersirable."[108] It does not require, however, that action B *will result* from the establishment of the precedent. Rather, it merely asserts that taking action A establishes a precedent such that action B *could* logically be accomplished.[109] It does not assert that action B *will* necessarily be accomplished.[110] The "undesirable consequence" established here—then—"is not a particular action B, but the presence of a precedent which would allow for other undesirable actions (possibly B, C, and D) if forces arose to pursue those actions."[111] Since suicide is a form of killing human life, it is arguable that it is morally similar to all other forms of killing human life and—furthermore—to either allow or condone it paves the way to the use of not only voluntary and involuntary euthanasia and infanticide, but other forms of destroying human life that might, under a given set of circumstances, be considered undesirable.[112]

To refute this position merely involves an understanding that suicide is the *voluntary* taking of *one's own life*, while infanticide is the involuntary taking of *another's life*. Thus, allowing suicide would not by any means establish an infanticide precedent. As to voluntary euthanasia—regarded as a type of "assisted" suicide—an argument could be maintained "that the involvement of another agent is morally relevant, and thus that allowing suicide would not establish a precedent for voluntary euthanasia."[113]

By acknowledging the suicide of an eighty year old woman in ill health is morally permissible would not necessarily establish a precedent for allowing the suicide of a twenty year old healthy woman. It might well set a precedent for allowing suicide in similar elderly people suffering from ill health. It should be stressed that not only are an individual's life *circumstances* morally relevant, but the *reasoning* advanced in support of an action is equally relevant to the establishment of a precedent.[114]

In sum, it is seen that on the basis of teleological reasoning it is improper to conclude that suicide is—in all cases—wrong. Under this basis of analysis, where an act of suicide results in more good than harm, it is right and not wrong.[115]

Deontological arguments have their bases not in assertions that suicide is wrong because it produces adverse consequences, but—rather—because the very act not only violates and degrades both the meaning and purpose of human life but destroys the very dignity of human nature.[116] Thus, the results of the action do not make it wrong, but rather something inherent in its nature. It is far beyond the purpose of this analysis to probe exhaustively the philosophical and ethical underpinnings of these deontological arguments against suicide—many of which duplicate and overlap. Suffice to mention in passing the major ones and select several for more probing analysis.

Suicide, it is argued, is unnatural and cowardly for it runs counter to the dignity of the person.[117] This in turn draws upon the Kantian thesis that all persons are ends in and of themselves and are held accountable to an absolute and universally applicable set of moral values and standards.[118] These moral arguments can be questioned as essentially but a series of unproven assumptions regarding the moral structure of the universe, the value of individual life as well as about refusals to take risks. These arguments are coupled with yet a further assumption of dubious generality: namely, that it is always wiser to err on the side of quantitative life than on standards of qualitative living.[119]

To judge suicide as a cowardly act is to, in reality, judge the actor's character—and not the action itself. An assessment of the character of the actor would only be relevant to judgments concerning moral *blameworthiness,* or when to assign blame or guilt, but not the *rightness* of an act.[120]

An act may be wrong but the actor blameworthy—for example, if there is some excusing condition or extenuating circumstance to explain why the actor did what she did. The assessment that an act was done out of cowardice does not, therefore, render the act wrong.[121]

Suicide is regarded as intrinsically wrong because it is an irrevocable act that prevents an individual's future quest for happiness.[122] This argument is obviously highly paternalistic and seeks to protect the long-term best interests of the at-risk individual,[123] and at the same time make an obviously premature or futuristic judgment about an individual's pursuit and obtainance of communal happiness over the long run. The future state of an individual's action is purely speculative at best. Indeed, since every action is based on an evaluation of certain probabilities that in turn foreclose future possibilities of one sort or another, this is an insufficient basis for suggesting a particular course of action should never be undertaken.[124]

It is argued that as a gift from God—life cannot be disposed of by humans, for suicide violates the commandment not to kill.[125] Since life *and* human freedom are co-equal gifts from God, lacking specific injunctions regarding the use of these gifts, "it is not clear that the giftedness of life *per se* constitutes an argument against suicide."[126] An unconventional approach to the "giftedness of life" argument would mandate no human intervention be taken at all throughout life—either to destroy or save it.[127] As to the biblical commandment argument, sophisticated biblical scholars are in agreement that the commandment not to kill should be interpreted as, "Thou shalt do no murder"—with "murder" being interpreted as not mere killing but wrongful killing.[128] Construed thusly, the controlling question is whether suicide is considered, under the individual facts of each case, murder (e.g., self murder) or wrongful killing.[129]

Finally, the deontologist argues that suicide is wrong because it is a renunciation of one's duty to himself to preserve his own life[130] and against a general duty to preserve life.[131] As to this Kantian assertion of a personal duty to oneself, it is suggested that a less cumbersome way of approaching this argument is to posture a re-definition of the concept of duty. Thus, those things which we have tended to call duties *to* oneself may actually be duties to others *regarding* oneself."[132] Accordingly, one may owe a duty to others to preserve his life, especially if he is the sole financial support of a family unit, but not a personal duty to self to preserve it.[133] With this re-interpretation, what is seen then is that this so-called duty to preserve one's life is more properly viewed as a general duty to mankind as a whole.[134]

This interpretation thus leads to the last argument that holds suicide is prohibitive because it derives from this generalized societal duty.[135] Accordingly, the view taken here is that suicide is wrong because—quite simply—it violates the principle of the sanctity or sacredness of all human life that holds life should never be taken directly by one's own actions or by others.[136] To adhere, logically, to such a position requires an opposition to *all* forms of destruction of human life, including capital punishment and "just" wars.[137] Interestingly, no such exceptionless stand is taken by most opponents of suicide.[138] "Unless the destruction of human life is to be condemned altogether, any principle by which some destruction of human life is permitted is likely to make room for at least some cases of suicide."[139]

What escapes the persuasiveness of the deontological and teleological arguments is that they neglect to recognize that as rational free moral agents, individuals should be respected in whatever choice of action they pursue in order to give their life meaning and substance—so long as that choice does not compromise the freedom of others. Regarding suicide, when individuals have chosen rationally to take their own lives—or in other words without coercion or under mental duress—and there are no overriding or contrary social-moral duties blocking this exercise of autonomy, they should be permitted to take their own lives without being censured or prohibited from exercising a morally "wrong" act. To posture this, does not mean that one is always morally *justified* in so acting. What it means is that one has a right to take his life "until a contravening moral obligation obtains."[140]

No doubt the most convincing reason against a recognition or condonation of suicide is that it compromises "certain *prima facie* duties of covenant fidelity—such as gratitude, promise-keeping, and reparations," one is thought of as owing to his family unit.[141] Again, in cases where there is no immediate family unit—parents, brothers and sisters, wife or children—it could be argued that such covenant duties are therefore non-existent and not binding on acts of self-determination such as suicide. What is seen in the final analysis, then, is that the root question of suicide or its "rightness" is tied to one of distributive justice—and, more specifically, of the achievement of a *balance* between the benefits of an individual's exercise of self-determination and personal good or satisfaction against the burdens, social obligations or claims of others that militate against such an act.[142]

Objections to the Use of Euthanasia

The central objections to the use of euthanasia parallel—to a very great degree—those raised regarding suicide. There are certain refinements that bear further analysis, however.

While recognizing the fact that death is not the greatest of all evils and that at some point in time "extreme measures of resistance are neither necessary nor appropriate,"[143] the concern has been expressed that increased interest and discussion of euthanasia is but a sad reflection of a spiritually bankrupt society.[144] What has been termed as a "contraceptive mentality," conditions the members of modern society to view life that is inconvenient as of no value and to seek its end through a merciful release.[145] Thus human choice is given greater purpose and direction than divine planning.[146] Stated otherwise, terminating life is violating God's property rights! Terming this objection as a form of "religious, biologistic determinism," that holds that organic collapse—or deterioration of the body and its processes—is the manner through which the will of God is manifested, would—taken to its logical extreme—paralyze the practice of medicine since, for example, by prescribing medicine, man's death is postponed.[147]

> Men who believe that God's will is manifested through the physical facts and events of life would have to sit back and await the good pleasure of nature. All efforts to step in and take over by reshaping the earth in accord with our own designs would be blasphemous.... The mentality of this objection is utterly at odds with genuine Christian theology. According to the Christian view, man is created in the image of the creator God. He is thus himself commissioned to creativity, a co-creator with God.... He is not a pawn of the earth's forces, but a participator in God's providence.... This, of course, is not to say that Christian theology is committed to death by choice. It is, however, to say that the presuppositions of the "playing God" objection are not Christian.... [148]

The Domino Theory or, never-forget-the-ghost-of-Nazi-Germany-and-the-Hollocaust, cautions that legalization of voluntary euthanasia would be but the first move to not only mass euthanasia but to genocide.[149] Fear, rather than rationality, is the operative force here.

The differences between contemporary American society and those of

Nazi Germany are of such dramatic significance that a simple and humane acceptance of voluntary euthanasia could never become the small beginning or wedge for a mass, and indiscriminate use of the act, itself. Several points substantiate this conclusion. First, the idea or principle of individual human rights—so inherent in modern society—had no place at all in Nazi Germany.[150] "Mercy killing for the benefit of the patient was not the point in Germany," and was rejected. People were killed because their life was deemed to be of no value to the German society."[151] The forced homogenity of the Nazi society does not exist in America today.[152] Indeed, various conflicting cultures both validate and strengthen pluralistic values.[153] Thus, before death by choice could ever become a national policy, extensive debate would be undertaken.[154] The Nazi experience has been so engrafted on the consciousness of contemporary society that this "deeply ingrained knowledge of human wickedness" serves as a strong symbol of a national resolve to exercise extreme caution in approaching and resolving issues of human, fundamental rights.[155]

Other salient concerns tie to the fact that if voluntary euthanasia were accepted, physicians would be but tools or servants to their patient's desire to end their lives;[156] that the possibility of an erroneous diagnosis of a patient's condition may mean a premature if not needless death;[157] that since modern pain relieving drugs mean an almost total elimination of pain (believed, by many, to be the worst aspect of dying), euthanasia should not be performed *carte blanche;*[158] and, finally, that the hope of a new medical discovery or surgical technique that would assist the incurable patient would be forthcoming.[159]

It is very difficult to imagine—short of financial coersion—how a physician would succumb to a patient's direction to administer euthanasia on demand. As presently structured, the ever-knowing fear of criminal prosecution for homicide or manslaughter would surely be a severe deterrent. That, plus professional censure, would hold in check the "mad" physician who might seek to hire himself out as a doctor of death. Erroneous diagnoses may be avoided by having a requirement enforced that directs an euthanee to be examined, and his prognosis confirmed by a panel of physicians. Although drugs are available to neutralize pain for most diseases (cancer of the throat and emphysema being notable exceptions), not only does the user suffer the problems of addition but—more importantly—harsh side effects to the usage such as unremitting vomiting, nausea and semiconsciousness. The lead time between the announcement by the Food and Drug Administration of a new "miracle" drug and its distribution can be significant enough to forestall reliance on an imminent miracle; similarly with new surgical techniques or technologies, years pass before they are ever approved or utilized widely.[160]

ENDNOTES

1. E.H. KLUGE, THE PRACTICE OF DEATH 131 (1975).

2. Laundau & Gustafson, Death Is Not The Enemy, 252 J.A.M.A. 2458 (1984).

3. Fried, The Value of Life in 1 ETHICAL, LEGAL AND SOCIAL CHALLENGES TO A BRAVE NEW WORLD, Ch. 1 (G. Smith ed. 1981).

4. Supra note 2.

5. Id.

6. E. BECKER, THE DENIAL OF DEATH 16, 17 (1973).

7. Id. at 51.

8. Fletcher, In Defense of Suicide in SUICIDE AND EUTHANASIA 38 at 48 (S. WALLACE, A. ESER eds. 1981).

9. D. MAGUIRE, DEATH BY CHOICE 156 (1975).

10. Id. at 157.

11. G. GRISEZ, J. M. BOYLE, JR., LIFE AND DEATH WITH LIBERTY AND JUSTICE 123, 124 (1979).

12. Supra note 8 at 49.

13. Smith, Quality of Life, Sanctity of Creation: Palliative or Apotheosis? 63 NEB. L. REV. 709 at 734, 735 (1984).

　　See also, Fletcher, Love is the Only Measure, 83 COMMONWEALTH 427 (1966).

14. See McCormick, To Save or Let Die: The Dilemma of Modern Medicine in HOW BRAVE A NEW WORLD 396 (R. McCormick ed. 1981).

15. Supra note 9 at 57.

16. Fletcher, Ethics and Euthanasia, 73 AM. J. NURSING 671 (1973).

17. Supra note 14 at 375.

18. Id.

19. Id. at 376, 377.

20. Id. at 328.

21. J. FLETCHER, HUMANHOOD: ESSAYS IN BIOMEDICAL ETHICS 167 (1979).

22. Id.

23. Id.

24. Id.

25. Id.

26. Id. at 168.

27. Id.

28. Id.

29. Id.

See generally, G. GRISEZ, J. B. BOYLE, JR., LIFE AND DEATH WITH LIBERTY AND JUSTICE Ch. 11 (1979).

If all individuals within a society can be regarded as having a *prima facie* obligation to treat people kindly, it could be argued that, as a kindness, beneficient euthanasia—or the painless inducement of a quick death that results in a benefit to the recipient—could be required of all. See M. KOHL, BENEFICIENT EUTHANASIA (1975).

30. GRISEZ & BOYLE, supra at 124.

31. Id.

The author maintains that the newly recognized "right" of privacy is nothing but certain aspects of liberty. Id. at 98.

32. Fletcher, In Defense of Suicide in SUICIDE AND EUTHANASIA: THE RIGHTS OF PERSONHOOD at 38, 50 (S. WALLACE, A. ESER eds. 1981).

33. G. Williams, Textbook of Criminal Law 579 (2d ed. 1983).

34. GRISEZ & BOYLE, supra note 29 at 127.

35. Id.

36. See Myers, Involuntary Civil Commitment for the Mentally Ill: A System in Need of Change, 29 VILL. L. REV. 367 (1983–84).

37. See e.g., *Bartling v. Superior Court*, 163 Cal. App. 3d 186, 209 Cal. Rptr. 220 (1984); *In re Hier*, 18 Mass. App. Ct. 200, 464 N.E. 2d 959 (1984); *In re Colyer*, 99 Wash. 2d 114, 600 P. 2d 738 (1983); *In re Eichner*, 73 A.D. 2d 431, 426 N.Y.S. 2d 517 (1980), *modified sub, nom., In re Storar*, 52 N.Y. 2d 363, 420 N.E. 2d 64, 438 N.Y.S. 2d 266 (1981).

38. Ladd, The Definition of Death and the Right to Die in ETHICAL ISSUES RELATING TO DEATH Ch. 6 at 129 (J. LADD ed. 1979).

39. Id. at 139.

See generally, R. FLATHMAN, THE PRACTICE OF RIGHTS (1976).

40. Supra note 38 at 139.

41. Id.

42. Id.

43. Id. at 140.

44. Jonas, The Right to Die, HASTINGS CENTER RPT. 31, 36 (Aug. 1978).

45. Id. at 34.

46. Id. at 35.

47. Ladd, Introduction, supra note 365 at 5.

48. Callahan, Autonomy: A Moral Good, Not a Moral Obsession, HASTINGS CENTER RPT. 40, 41 (Oct. 1984).

49. Id.

50. Id.

51. Id.

52. Id.

53. Id.

54. Id. at 42.

55. The Six Great Humanistic Essays of John Stuart Mill, On Liberty, Ch. 1, Introduction, at 135 (A. Levi, ed. 1969).

56. Id.

See T. BEAUCHAMP, J. CHILDRESS, PRINCIPLES OF BIOMEDICAL ETHICS, Ch. 3 (2d ed. 1983).

57. Veatch, Autonomy's Temporary Triumph, HASTINGS CENTER RPT. 38 (Oct. 1984).

58. Morrison, The Biological Limits on Autonomy, HASTINGS CENTER REPORT 43 (Oct. 1984).

59. Appelbaum & Klein, Therefore Choose Death? 12 HUMAN LIFE REV. 100 (1986).

60. Id. at 104.

61. Id.

62. Id.

63. Id. at 103.

64. Id. at 109.

See also, Smith, *Triage:* Endgame Realities, 1 J. CONTEMP. HEALTH L. & POL'Y 143 (1985).

65. Id. at 108.

66. Stone, Judges as Medical Decision Makers, HUMAN LIFE REV. 84, 88 (1986).

67. Shultz, From Informed Consent to Patient Choice: A New Protected Interest, 95 YALE L. J. 219 (1985).

68. Id.

69. Id.

See generally, McCormick & Veatch, The Prolongation of Life and Self-Determination, 41 THEOLOGICAL STUDIES 390 (1980).

70. Supra note 67 at 221.

71. Id.

72. Id. at 222.

73. Id.

74. Id.

75. Id. at 223, 275, 276.

76. Id. at 278.

77. Id. at 284, 285.

78. Id. at 299.

79. Id.

80. Shultz, From Informed Consent to Patient Choice: A New Protected Interest, 95 YALE L.J. 219, 299 (1985).

81. C. Fried, Right or Wrong 146–147 (1978).

See generally Jackson & Younger, Patient Autonomy and "Death with Dignity," 301 NEW ENG. J. MED. 404 (1979).

82. J. CHILDRESS, WHO SHOULD DECIDE? PATERNALISM IN HEALTH CARE 13 (1982).

83. Id. at 13.

84. Id. at 2.

85. Id. at Ch. 5.

86. Id. at 105.

87. Id. at 109.

88. Id.

89. Newman, Treatment Refusals for the Critically and Terminally Ill: Proposed Rules for the Family, The Physician and the State, 3 N.Y. L. SCH. HUMAN RIGHTS ANN. 35 (1985).

90. Id.

91. Id. at 62.

92. Id. at 61.

93. Id.

94. Id. at 62.

Many physicians need to feel dominant and in control. J. KATZ, THE SILENT WORLD OF DOCTOR AND PATIENT, n. 107 at 148–149 (1984).

95. Lebacqz & Englehardt, Suicide in DEATH, DYING AND EUTHANASIA at 669, 673 (D. HORAN, D. MALL eds. 1977).

96. Id.

97. Id.

98. Id. at 674.

99. Id.

100. Id.

See also, R. BRANDT, ETHICAL THEORY 106, 182 (1959).

101. Baelz, Voluntary Euthanasia: Some Theological Reflections, 75 THEOLOGY 238, 244 (1959).

102. Supra note 95 at 675.

103. Id.

104. Id.

105. Id. at 676.

106. Id.

107. Id.

See also, Childress, Who Shall Live When Not All Can Live? 43 SOUNDINGS 339 (1970).

108. Id. at 677.

109. Id. at 678.

110. Id.

111. Id.

112. Id.

See Arros, The Right to Die on the Slippery Slope, 8 SOCIAL THEORY & PRACTICE 285 (Fall 1982).

113. Id. at 680.

114. Id.

115. Id.

116. Id. at 681.

117. Id. at 680–682.

118. E. KLUGE, THE PRACTICE OF DEATH 141 (1975).

119. Id. at 147.

120. Lebacqz & Englehardt, Suicide in DEATH, DYING AND EUTHANASIA at 682 (D. HORAN, D. MALL eds. 1977).

121. Id.
122. Id. at 622.
123. Id.
124. Id. at 683.
125. Id. at 685.
126. Id.
127. Id.
128. Id.
129. Id. at 686.
    The definition of suicide as murder can only have efficacy if an act of murder is sought to be defined a direct and intentional killing of an innocent human life—independent of any consideration of what determines the wrongness of murder and whether, as a consequence of this, a taking of human life may be justified under some circumstances. "If the evil in murder is the radical subversion of another's freedom, then it is morally significant when the actor and the 'victim' are the same—i.e., when no one's freedom is being subverted. In short, what holds *prima facie* in the case of taking the life of another may not hold in the case of taking one's life." It has been suggested that "if suicide is murder then 'by parity of reasoning, marriage is really adultery—' own wife 'adultery.'" Id.
130. Id. at 687.
131. Id. at 688.
132. Id. at 687.
133. Id.
134. Id.
135. Id. at 688.
136. Id.
    See M. KOHL, THE MORALITY OF KILLING 3 (1974).
137. Id.
138. Id.
139. Id.
140. Id. at 689.
141. Id. at 690.
142. E. KULGE, THE PRACTICE OF DEATH 289, 292 (1975).
143. C. RICE, BEYOND ABORTION: THE THEORY AND THE PRACTICE IN A SECULAR STATE 119 (1979).
144. Id. at 129.
145. Id.
146. D. MAGUIRE, DEATH BY CHOICE 141 (1975).
147. Id. at 142.
148. Id. at 143.
149. Id. at 131, 132.
150. Id. at 134.
151. Id.
152. Id.
153. Id.

154. Id.

155. Id.

See generally, R. VEATCH, DEATH, DYING AND THE BIOLOGICAL REVOLUTION, Ch. 3 (1976), for a discussion of the pro and con arguments regarding euthanasia; Louisell, Euthanasia and Bianthanisia: On Dying and Killing, 22 CATH. U.L. REV. 723, 742 (1973).

156. J. CHILDRESS, WHO DECIDES? PATERNALISM IN HEALTH CARE 178 (1982).

157. Kamisar, Some Proposed Non-Religious Views Against Proposed Mercy Killing Legislation, 42 MINN. L. REV. 469 (1958).

158. Supra note 156 at 179.

See also, Sharma, Euthanasia in Australasia, 2 J. CONTEMP. HEALTH L. & POL'Y 131, 145 (1986).

159. Sharma, supra at 143.

160. Id. at 146.

Chapter III

PERSONHOOD AND THE CONCEPT OF PERSON

COMPETENCY V. INCOMPETENCY

To be treated as a person, one must not only enjoy states of consciousness as well as intentional states, have the capacity to have experiences which occur at different times and are linked together by memory[1] or—stated otherwise—have a capacity for love and engaging in interpersonal relationships (or, what has been termed the "relational potential").[2] Whether rationality or social interactive capacities are the controlling criteria to establish personhood remains an open philosophical question. It has been suggested that an individual's moral standing as part of the moral community should be permitted to end only when a reasonable deduction can be made that a clear breakdown in linkage between bodily integrity and mental or social capacity is established.[3]

In order to assist in determining when life may be terminated from a point of moral justification, various questions may be posited.[4] Nine of the most relevant ones are: 1.) Is the individual in question characterized as a person? 2.) If it is so characterized, does it desire its own death—and if this is the case, is that a rational desire? 3.) If the person is sustained, what quality of life will be enjoyed? 4.) What are the economic costs of maintaining this person's life? 5.) Is the person in an unconscious state and technologically impossible of being restored to consciousness? 6.) Would the termination of life be a matter of active intervention or but a matter of exercising restraint in saving the person's life? 7.) Is the case in point one involving direct or indirect "killing"? 8.) Does the action contemplated require "extraordinary" or only "ordinary" means in order to maintain the person alive? 9.) Is the nature of the illness suffered by the individual *in extremis* of a fatal nature?[5]

Another complementary framework for helpful analysis has been set out as so-called indicators of "humanhood" which, it is thought, when evaluated provide a profile of some fifteen qualities or attitudes regarded as necessary for one to be regarded as a "person." Among the indicators are:

self-awareness; self-control; time consciousness; a sense of futurity; a sense of memory; a capability to relate to others; an ability to communicate; the ability to assert control and not display utter helplessness; the ability to display curiosity instead of indifference; rationality; the ability to be emotive and intuitive; and—finally—the capacity for neo-cortial functions.[6]

> In the absence of the synthesizing function of the cerebral cortex, the *person* is non-existent. Such individuals are objects not subjects.... Personal reality depends on cerebration and to be dead "humanly" speaking is to be ex-cerebral, no matter how long the body remains alive.[7]

What both the nine questions posted previously regarding the point at which life may be terminated and the indicators of humanhood have in common is the shared focus upon the brain and its proper functioning as the key to the advancement or—as the case may be—the preclusion of all of the complex human responses and attitudes which tend toward identifying and recognizing a human as a functioning person.

TOWARD A UNIFORM DETERMINATION OF DEATH?

The traditional legal definition of death has been, "The cessation of life; permanent cessation of all vital functions and signs."[8] As to the determination of death, from a biological standpoint, the law has treated the matter—generally—as a question of medical fact, determined according to those criteria established by the medical profession in each state;[9] and consequently no consensus is to be found among the states regarding the matter. Limited application of a brain death standard has been authorized by thirty-three states, with twenty-seven states having codified brain death statutes and[10] the remaining six validating brain death determination by judicial cognizance.[11]

State legislative approaches to determining death may be grouped into a three pong classification. The first pong consists of seven states which have chosen to flow an "alternative" approach—providing as such that the occurrence of death will be recognized when a patient suffers an irreversible cessation of spontaneous cardiorespiratory function or sustains irreversible cessation of spontaneous brain function.[12] It is obvious that this approach allows for a perception—inaccurate though it may be— that there is a recognition of two entirely different phenomena of death.[13]

The second prong is found among eight states and, while providing for alternative standards for determining death, is careful to elucidate the specific conditions under which each standard is to be applied.[14] Typically, these statutes provide that death is recognized legally when there is an irreversible cessation of cardiorespiratory function—unless respiration and heart beat are maintained by means of artificial support, in which case death occurs when the brain function is determined to be irreversible.[15]

Finally, the third prong has been developed and applied in twelve states by legislative enactment, and applies a brain death standard for determining the occurrence of death.[16] Within this group, some legislative directions require irreversible cessation of brain functions in order to determine death and thus recognize a strictly exclusive standard of brain death;[17] while other statutes require that death be recognized when there is an irreversible cessation of brain function, yet go further and allow the use of other medically accepted standards in determining death.[18]

By dictating exclusive reliance upon brain death as the determiner of death, a physician is effectively precluded from letting the circumstances of each individual case tie to ordinary medical procedures used for determining death. Statutes of this nature also preclude necessary flexibility being utilized where the state of the medical technology is such that new, more effective advances might eclipse a traditional brain death standard and be necessary to be implemented in order to allow for the harvesting of vital organs for critical transplant surgeries.

In 1968, in an effort to assist themselves as a profession, and the law as well, to seek some degree of uniformity in the area of death, a number of physicians at the Harvard Medical School issued a report which established four criteria for the diagnosis of irreversible coma:[19] unreceptivity and unresponsivity to externally applied stimuli and inner need; no spontaneous muscular movements or spontaneous respiration; no elicitable brain reflexes and a flat EEG or electroencephalogram.[20] The report also suggested that in a case where findings of this type were made, a subsequent verification of them be undertaken at least twenty-four hours later. It was furthermore suggested that, upon the fulfillment of the criteria, and before any effort was undertaken to disconnect a respirator, the patient be officially declared dead.[21] The Committee's Report was not presented for the purpose of replacing the more traditional standards for determining death; on the contrary, they were urged only as a complement.[22]

In 1981, Dr. William Street, a member of the original medical committee that wrote the Harvard Brain Death Criteria, observed that, in actual implementation, the Criteria has been found to be too strict as to some, and too lax as to others. Of particular concern to him was the fact that the criteria fails to make an adequate distinction between irreversible coma and brain death. He did note that there are no present records disclosing any recovery for patients who met the criteria.[23]

The National Conference of Commissioner's of Uniform State Laws approved in 1978 The Uniform Brain Death Act that states:

> For legal and medical purposes, an individual who has sustained irreversible cessation of all functioning of the brain, including the brain stem is dead. A determination under this section must be made in accordance with reasonable medical standards.[24]

Before this Act was superseded in 1980 by the Commissioners' adoption of The Uniform Determination of Death Act, four states passed legislation adopting its original provisions.[25]

The President's Commission for the Study of Ethical Problems in Medicine and Biomedical and Behavioral Research concluded in 1981 that the states should adopt a model statute entitled, "The Uniform Determination of Death Act," which would establish much needed clarity and certainty.[26] Under this statute,

> An individual who has sustained either (1) irreversible cessation of circulatory and respiratory functions or (2) irreversible cessation of all functions of the entire brain, including the brain stem, is dead. A determination of death must be made in accordance with accepted medical standards.[27]

Since the issuance of this Report and its recommendation and the subsequent approval by the National Conference of Commissioners on Uniform State Laws in August, 1980, of this Uniform Act, it has been adopted legislatively in fifteen states and the District of Columbia[28] and judicially in two."[29]

Interestingly, public acceptance of the concept of brain death has not been uniform; for the average, ordinary person still perceives stoppage of the heart as the sole determinant of death.[30] With time, however, and more dramatic "real life" news coverage of tragic Karen Quinlan-type cases, the public will hopefully become more aware, and thus possibly more fully educated on this matter.[31]

A very meritorious and, indeed, persuasive suggestion has been offered as a means of resolving the present confusion and controversy over standards for defining death—specifically, the adoption of neocortical death as the operative and controlling medico-legal standard.[32] Defining this type of death as "the irreversible loss of consciousness and cognitive function,"[33] the present legal inconsistency of upholding surrogate decisions to terminate life-support systems together with nourishment when incompetent patients irreversibly lose all consciousness and cognitive functions—yet failing to recognize neocortical death—is observed.[34] It is then submitted that if this type of death were legally validated, the moral and legal dilemmas inherent within this area of consideration would be resolved in very large part because once a physician has made a determination that a patient had lost, irreversibly, all cerebral qualities of human life, the patient would be recognized as legally dead and—thus—artificial life supports, together with nourishment, could be terminated. Substituted judgment and best interest tests would no longer be required in order to *guess* what course of treatment or non-treatment should be pursued.[35]

While preeminently reasonable, this suggestion is somewhat ahead of its time for social acceptance. Wrenching though the tragic choice are regarding a continuance of "life" or a passive act of cessation of it, this unduly full and open process has a cathartic effect on all parties—and especially the system of justice that forswears equality of treatment for all within a forum of open family debate and hoped-for concensus. Put quite simply, oh too many people *feel* that so long as there is breath, there is life and would surely feel uncomfortable about the utilization of this abrupt, albeit merciful, standard of neo-cortical death. To compound the "public relations" matter here is the fact that those who are brain dead still are capable of spontaneous and cardiac respiratory functioning. Indeed, adult patients—declared brain dead—may give every appearance of life and especially so to those (members of the family) unfamiliar with such technologies as mechanical ventilation and total parenteral nutrition. The average family involved here has time and time again shown that abrupt and final decisions that would be allowed by adoption and application of the neo-cortical standard of death are not acceptable to their feelings. Agonizing though such decisions are, given the average unsophistication of the dying and the fear of death, much education will have to be undertaken to prepare the ordinary American for acceptance of this standard as well as brain death in general.

LIVING WILLS AND NATURAL DEATH ACTS

A so-called "living will" is an instrument that indicates its maker's preference not to be started or maintained on a course of extraordinary treatment (sometimes specific modalities are designated) in the event of accidental or debilitating illness.[36] The biggest uncertainty surrounding living wills and their subsequent administration is related to whether health care providers are required—under pain of civil or criminal sanction—to execute the terms of the will. An interlinking concern is whether those participants charged with fulfilling the terms of the will be assured of immunity from civil or criminal prosecution.[37] Whether a refusal of life sustaining therapies would constitute a suicide remains largely as yet another vexatious and unresolved issue.[38] Regardless of these points of great uncertainty, some thirty-five states and the District of Columbia have passed living will legislation.[39]

Those jurisdictions recognizing living wills are faced with the fact that they must still address the issue of the nature of the medical techniques they will determine to be "extraordinary" and the type of circumstances which will "demonstrate that the person's previously expressed desire to forego treatment continued up to the time immediately prior to his or her disability."[40] Without legislative decisions that tackle forthrightly and with clarity these issues, the courts will be faced with a case-by-case determination of the parameters of life.[41]

In an effort to correct some of the weaknesses and uncertainties of living will legislation, more and more states are enacting Natural Death Acts.[42] Spurred by California's bold and innovative effort in 1976 in passing a Natural Death Act designed to formally establish the requirements for a "directive to physicians," other states have begun to follow suit and authorize validly executed instruments relieving a physician, staff and hospital from civil and criminal liability for removing or withholding life-sustaining treatments.[43] Considerable difference exists among the various legislative programs regarding the assessment of penalties for either disobeying the directive of a properly executed instrument or preventing the transfer of a patient seeking to come within the provisions of the law to another physician who will respect and follow the patient's wishes.[44] And, the triggering mechanisms of the legislation are often cumbersome and self-defeating. In California, for example, before a patient may seek to avail himself of the provisions of The Natural Death Act, he must first receive a diagnosis as being in a terminal condition which is construed as meaning "an incurable condition with death being imminent regardless of life-sustaining procedures.[45]

In actual practice, there is evidence to suggest that a patient's ability to have his wishes regarding the prohibition of life-sustaining treatment may be impeded in states where Natural Death legislation exists.[46] For, if such legislation is viewed by attending physicians and health care providers as the sole means for both initiating and implementing a decision to forego treatment and if a further belief is maintained that a decision of this nature cannot be made by a surrogate on behalf of another but only in strict accordance with an advance directive that has been executed properly by a patient, dying patients may in fact be subject to treatment the nature of which is neither requested nor beneficial.[47] There is additional fear that an improper inference may be drawn that if a patient has not executed a directive that is in compliance with natural death legislation, he does not wish methods of life sustaining treatment to be *ended* under any and all circumstances.[48] The truth of the matter might well reveal that a directive was not executed because of either ignorance of its legislative existence, an unawareness of its importance or even uncertainty regarding how it should be composed.[49]

Generally, the right to die or natural death acts apply only to "competent adults,"[50] with children and those mentally incompetent being excluded. Yet, some jurisdictions have made provision for proxy consent. In North Carolina, the controlling statute allows proxy consent for an irreversibly comatose patient who has not previously executed a living will—with consent being given by a spouse, legal guardian or a majority of the relatives of the first degree.[51] No reference is made in the statute to any other type of incompetent patient. Virginia legislation does not expressly allude to the rights of patients with inadequate decision making capacity and refers only to competent patients.[52] In New Mexico, provision is made for proxy consent for minors—although not for incompetent adults.[53] Arkansas legislation, however, covers both minors and incompetent adults, alike.[54]

DURABLE POWERS OF ATTORNEY

As a consequence of the numerous weaknesses encountered with Living Will legislation and Natural Death Acts, it has been suggested that additional safeguards should be utilized for implementing advance directions on life sustaining modalities of treatment. Specifically, adoption of proxy directives through durable powers of attorney statutes would go far toward assuring an individual's desires regarding treatment (or, as the case may be, non-treatment) would be effected.[55] Forty-two states have enacted laws authorizing durable powers of attorney that enable the appointment of a proxy to act after a person becomes incompetent.[56] The language of these statutes is usually broad enough to accommodate the appointment of a surrogate to facilitate problems which involve health care for the incompetent—although the statutes were not enacted for remedying these specific problems of incompetence, however.[57]

Since the usual power of attorney—which may be either of general or limited nature—ceases when the principal becomes incapacitated, some states have created specific durable powers of attorneys whereby an agent's authority to act is specifically mandated to continue after a debilitating event happens to the principal.[58] In this way, the power may be used as an "advance proxy directive" whereby an individual can nominate another whose express duty it will be to make *all* decisions regarding health care in the event the principal becomes incapacitated or otherwise unable to make decisions of that nature.[59] As can be seen, this advances greatly the efficiency and fairness of the whole decision making process for incapacitated persons.

As durable power of attorney statutes begin to be adapted and applied to areas to which they were not originally designed to accommodate, care and study must be undertaken to make certain these original procedures—initially enacted to "avoid the expense of full guardianship or conservatorship proceedings when dealing with small property interests"—are not abused in cases of application to incapacitated patients.[60] At some point in time, procedural safeguards may well have to be designed in order to assure necessary and functional application of the durable powers of attorney. There is no question, however, of their great potential and their already proven success in easing the heavy and emotional burdens of decision making here and their added value in allowing the courts to respect individual and familial privacy by not intruding.[61]

A STATUTORY CLARIFICATION?

In August, 1985, the National Conference of Commissioners on Uniform State Laws approved and recommended for enactment in all the states a Uniform Rights of the Terminally Ill Act.[62] This Act authorizes an adult to execute a declaration to his physicians and health care facilities directing the withholding or withdrawing of life-sustaining treatment in the event he is in a terminal condition of health and thereby unable to participate in decisions concerning medical treatment. The scope of the Act is quite narrow in that it but provides *one* way for the wishes of a terminally ill person regarding the use of life-sustaining procedures to be fulfilled. It is designed to avoid inconsistency in approach to decision making here which has continued to plague living will statutes by providing simply that the effectiveness of such a statutory declaration will be executed uniformly in all states other than the one in which it is made.

The Act is not intended to affect any existing rights and responsibilities of persons to make medical treatment decisions. Furthermore, its provisions are limited to treatment that is merely life prolonging and to those patients whose terminal condition is incurable and/or irreversible, whose death will soon occur and who are unable to participate in medical treatment decisions. It does not address issues of the treatment of persons who have not executed a statutory declaration of this nature nor does it pertain to treatment issues for minors nor treatment decisions made by proxy. Although drawing upon the basic structure and substance of similar existing living will legislation, it simplifies procedures, improves drafting and clarifies language such as the terms "life sustaining treatment"[63] and "terminal condition."[64] Legislation of this type that endeavors to clarify terms and concepts in this critical area of concern must be applauded as a positive action. It of course remains to be seen whether the states view the model as a clarification or an obfuscation.[65]

THE HEMLOCK SOCIETY INITIATIVE

The Hemlock Society of California is presently undertaking a campaign to place as a referendum initiative an amendment to the State Constitution that would recognize and expand "the inalienable right of privacy" to include "the right of the terminally ill to voluntary, humane, and dignified doctor assisted aid in dying."[66] The subsequent Act emerging from this proposed amendment is termed the Humane and Dignified Death Act and structures a mechanism that would allow adults to,

> ... execute a directive directing the withholding or withdrawal of life-sustaining procedures or, if suffering from a terminal condition, administering aid in dying. The directive shall be signed by the declar-

ant in the presence of two witnesses not related to the declarant by blood or marriage and who would not be entitled to any portion of the estate of the declarant upon his death under any will of the declarant or codicil thereto then existing or, at the time of the directive, by operation of law then existing. In addition, a witness to a directive shall not be the attending physician, an employee of the attending physician or a health care facility in which the declarant is a patient, nor any person who, at the time of the execution of the directive, has a claim against any portion of the estate of the declarant upon his death.[67]

For declarants who are patients in a "skilled nursing facility" to make a valid directive, one of the two witnesses must in fact be a patient advocate or ombudsman designated as such by the California State Department of Aging.[68] Provision is made for the revocation of the directive by the declarant "without regard to his mental state or competency"[69] and an exculpatory clause prohibits an imposition of "criminal, civil or administrative liability on the part of any person for failure to act upon a revocation . . . unless that person has actual knowledge of the revocation."[70]

No civil, criminal or administrative liability is imposed upon a physician or licensed health professional acting under the direction of a physician who fails, "to effectuate the directive of the qualified patient . . . unless he wilfully fails to transfer the patient to a physician who will comply with the directive."[71] More specifically, actions of withholding "or withdrawal" of life-sustaining procedures from or administering aid in dying to a qualified patient," under this Act will not be regarded as acts of suicide.[72] Provision is made for amending the Civil Code, Section 2443, by providing that actions under the Humane and Dignified Death Act shall not be construed as condoning, authorizing or approving mercy killing or permitting "any affirmative or deliberate act or omission to end life other than the withholding or withdrawal of health care pursuant to a durable power of attorney for health care so as to permit the natural process of dying."[73] The proposed amendment to Section 2443 of the Civil Code makes it clear that, "an attempted suicide by the principal shall not be construed to indicate a desire of the principal that health care treatment be restricted or inhibited or that aid in dying be given."[74] It should be stressed that the Proposed Act does not condone, authorize or approve mercy killing or permit any affirmative or deliberate act or omission to end life *other than* by a licensed physician and when requested by the patient pursuant to a properly executed legal document.

The Model Directive proposed by the Hemlock Society to accompany this proposed legislation in Article Two states:

> In the absence of my ability to give directions regarding the termination of my life, it is my intention that this directive shall be honored by my family, agent and physician(s) as the final expression of my legal right to 1) REFUSE MEDICAL OR SURGICAL TREATMENT and 2) TO CHOOSE TO DIE IN A HUMANE AND DIGNIFIED MANNER.

Provision is made in Article Three that if a diagnosis of pregnancy is made and known by the physician, the directive will have neither force or effect during the course of the pregnancy.

Article Four stipulates the declarant's understanding that he has a terminal illness for which it is not likely he will live with treatment *more than six months.* In Article Five, the declarant's agent is given "full power and authority to make health care decisions" to the same extent as the declarant would if capacitated. In exercising this authority, the agent is required to make those decisions consistent with the declarant's desires as specified in the directive "or otherwise made known" to the agent "including, but not limited to" the desires of the declarant "concerning obtaining or refusing or withdrawing life-prolonging care, treatment, services and procedures, and administration of aid in dying."

The Humane and Dignified Death Initiative is an eloquent effort to build upon the Living Will legislation, Natural Death Acts and durable powers of attorney acts to finally recognize—in a definitive legislative scheme—that the continuation of life for terminally ill persons under conditions of severe pain and suffering constitutes not only severe cruelty and disregard for human dignity but an invasion into basic rights of privacy and self-determination. It can be but hoped that the Humane and Dignified Death Initiative sponsored by the Hemlock Society will in fact be accepted by the citizens of California and, as such, begin to structure a framework for principled national decision-making in this central area of human values and ethical concerns.[75]

NEW BEGINNINGS?

From this analysis, it can be seen and understood that—modernly—death cannot be identified easily as one event or configuation; for the very gradualness of it as a process can be apprehended when it is realized that multiple parts of the body can continue to live even after the disintegration of its central organization is recorded.[76] Indeed, more and more, man's physiological system does not collapse and fail in a moment's time. Rather, technological substitutes are capable of use and total integration by a wondrously "evil" computer. Thus, while the vital signs are evidenced, they are both provided and manipulated by machines.

These various new medical-legal approaches to aid definitions of death have one great practical merit however: they endeavor to place and to recognize the moment of death earlier in the continuum of life than did earlier practice and definitional structure. And, in so doing, the physician's decision to discontinue therapy even though what were regarded commonly as "signs of life" are nevertheless present, is made considerably easier. Death may then come with dignity and often mercy. Not only does this disallow the immediate and extended family members, as well as attending health care providers, with the deep anguish of dealing with a living corpse, but also preclude the assessment of heavy economic burdens of caring for one who has lost the basic attributes or indicators of personhood. Additionally, the body parts that survive death—as thus newly classified and defined—may be harvested and made available to deserving recipients without the physicians being fearful and uncertain that their acts might be considered invasions of privacy or criminal assaults.[77]

The Emerging Construct

The construct for principled decision making here is one obviously being structured partially in legislative enactments of the nature thus analyzed. These enactments bear clear and unmistakable evidence that complex social mechanisms of the day are at force in re-establishing and asserting the right of every individual to autonomy and enlightened self-determination in deciding his final rite of passage. Passive euthanasia and rational suicide are offensive words of parlance of a time long gone by. Autonomy and enlightened self-determination are the more contemporaneous watch-words of today.

ENDNOTES

1. Tooley, Decisions to Terminate Life and The Concept of Persons in ETHICAL ISSUES RELATING TO LIFE AND DEATH at 85–87 (J. LADD ed. 1979).

2. McCormick, To Save, or Let Die: The Dilemmas of Modern Medicine in HOW BRAVE A NEW WORLD? at 339–349 (R. McCormick ed. 1981).

3. R. VEATCH, A THEORY OF MEDICAL ETHICS 240–244, at 245 (1981).

4. Id. Professor Tooley lists thirteen such questions. Supra note 1.

5. Supra note 1 at 62, 63.

6. Fletcher, Indicators of Humanhood: A Tentative Profile of Man, 13 HASTINGS CENTER RPT. 1 (Nov. 1972).

7. Id. at 3.

8. BLACK'S LAW DICTIONARY 360 (5th ed. 1979).

In an article entitled, "On Defining a 'Natural Death,'" Daniel Callahan has attempted to provide a stipulative definition of "Natural Death" thusly: "the individual event of death at that point in a life span when (a) one's life work has been accomplished; (b) one's moral obligations to those for whom one has had responsibility have been discharged; (c) one's death will not seem to others as offense to sense or sensibility, or tempt others to despair and rage at human existence; and finally (d) one's process of dying is not marked by unbearable and degrading pain." HASTINGS CENTER RPT. 33 (June 1977).

9. See Brennan & Delgado, Death: Multiple Definitions or a Single Standard?, 54 SO. CAL. L. REV. 1323 (1981); Dornette, How Does Your State Define Death?, 8 LEGAL ASPECTS MED. PRAC. 19 (No. 5, 1980).

See also, High, Is "Natural Death" an Illusion? HASTINGS CENTER RPT. 37 (Aug. 1978) where the author suggests the central concern should not be directed to determining natural death, but rather three more critical issues: the right to refuse treatment; an analysis of whether or not a particular treatment is—as to each individual case—medically indicated; and what standards are needed to assure proper care for the dying in order that they may die with dignity. Id. at 42.

10. See ALA. CODE §22-33-1 to -4 (1984); ALASKA STAT. §09.65.120 (1983); ARK. STAT. ANN. §82-537 (Supp. 1983); CAL. HEALTH & SAFETY CODE §7180 (West Supp. 1985); CONN. GEN. STAT. ANN. §19-139(i)(b) (1977); FLA. STAT. ANN. §382.085 (Supp. 1985); GA. CODE ANN. §88-1715.1 (1979); HAWAII REV. STAT. §327C-1 (Supp. 1984); IDAHO CODE §54-1819 (Supp. 1985); ILL. ANN. STAT. ch. 110, §302(b) (Smith-Hurd 1985); IOWA CODE §702.8 (1979); KAN. STAT. ANN. §77-205 (1984); LA. REV. STAT. ANN. §9:111 (West Supp. 1985); MD. ANN. CODE §5-202 (1984 Supp.); MICH. COMP. LAWS §333.1021 (1980); MISS. CODE ANN. §41-36-3 (1981); MONT. CODE ANN. §50-22-101 (1983); NEV. REV. STAT. §451.007 (1979); N.M. STAT. ANN. §12-2-4 (1978); N.C. GEN. STAT. §90-323 (1981); OKLA. STAT. ANN. tit. 63, §1-301(g) (1984); OR. REV. STAT. §146.001 (1983); TENN. CODE ANN. §53-459 (1982 Supp.); TEX. REV. CIV. STAT. ANN., art. 4447t (Vernon Supp. 1981); VA. CODE §54-325.7 (1982 Supp.); W. VA. CODE §16-10-2 (1985); WYO. STAT. §35-19-101 (Supp. 1985).

11. See *Arizona v. Fierro*, 124 Ariz. 182, 603 P. 2d 74, 77–78 (1979) (adoption of Uniform Brain Death Act); *Lovato v. District Court*, 198 Colo. 418, 601 P. 2d 1072, 1081 (1979) (adoption of Uniform Brain Death Act); *Swafford v. State*, _____ Ind. _____, 421 N.E. 2d 596, 602 (1981) (adoption of Uniform Determination of Death Act); Commonwealth v. Golston, 373 Mass. 249, 366 N.E. 2d 744, 748–49 (1977) (adoption of brain death standard), *cert. denied*, 434 U.S. 1039 (1978); *New York City Health & Hosp. Corp. v. Sulsona*, 81 Misc. 2d 1002, 1007, 367 N.Y.S. 2d 686, 691 (Sup. Ct. 1975)

(adoption of brain death standard for transplantation purposes); *In re Welfare of Bowman,* 94 Wash. 2d 407, 421, 617 P. 2d 731, 738 (1980) (adoption of Uniform Determination of Death Act).

12. IDAHO CODE §54-1819 (Supp. 1981) (Uniform Determination of Death Act); KAN. STAT. ANN. §77-202 (Supp. 1981); MD. ANN. CODE, art. 43, §54F (1980); MISS. CODE ANN. §41-36-3 (1981) (Uniform Determination of Death Act); N.M. STAT. ANN. §12-2-4 (1978); OR. REV. STAT. §146.001 (Supp. 1981); VA. CODE §54-325.7 (Supp. 1980).

13. See Capron & Kass, A Statutory Definition of the Standards for Determining Human Death: An Appraisal and a Proposal, 121 U. PA. L. REV. 87, 109 (1972).

14. See ALA. CODE §22-31-1 (Supp. 1981); ALASKA STAT. §09.65.120 (Supp. 1981); FLA. STAT. ANN. §382.085 (Supp. 1981); HAWAII REV. STAT. §327C-1 (Supp. 1979); IOWA CODE §702:8 (1979); LA. REV. STAT. ANN. §9:111 (West Supp. 1981); MICH. COMP. LAWS §333.102 (1980); TEX. REV. CIV. STAT. ANN. art. 4447t (Vernon Supp. 1981).

15. Id.

16. See ARK. STAT. ANN. §82-537 (Supp. 1981); CAL. HEALTH & SAFETY CODE §7180 (West Supp. 1981); CONN. GEN. STAT. §19-139i(b) (West Supp. 1981); GA. CODE ANN. §88-1715 (1979); ILL. ANN. STAT. ch. 110½ §302(b) (Smith-Hurd 1978) (only applies to UAGA); MONT. REV. CODE ANN. §50-22-101 (1979); NEV. REV. STAT. §451.007 (1979) (Uniform Brain Death Act); N.C. GEN. STAT. §90-323 (1981); OKLA. STAT. ANN. tit. 63 §1-301(g) (West Supp. 1981); TENN. CODE ANN. §54-459 (1977); W. VA. CODE §16-10-2 (Supp. 1981), (Uniform Brain Death Act); WYO. STAT. §35-19-101 (Supp. 1981).

17. See ARK. STAT. ANN. §82-537 (Supp. 1981); ILL. ANN. STAT. ch. 110½ §302(b) (Smith-Hurd 1978); MONT. REV. CODE ANN. §50-22-101 (1979); NEV. REV. STAT. §451.007 (1979); OKLA. STAT. ANN. tit. 63, §1-301(g) (West Supp. 1981); TENN. CODE ANN. §53-459 (1977); W. VA. CODE §16-10-2 (Supp. 1981); WYO. STAT. §35-19-101 (Supp. 1981).

18. See CAL. HEALTH & SAFETY CODE §7180 (West Supp. 1981); CONN. GEN. STAT. ANN. §19-139(i)(b) (West Supp. 1981); GA. CODE ANN. §88-1717 (1979); N.C. GEN. STAT. §90-323 (1981).

     See also, *State v. Fierro,* 124 Ariz. 182, 603 P. 2d 74, 77–79 (1979) (common law definition still sufficient to establish death despite adoption of brain death standard); *Lovato v. District Court,* 198 Colo. 418, 601 P. 2d 1072, 1081 (1979) (adoption of Uniform Brain Death Act does not preclude continuing recognition of common law standard).

19. A Definition of Irreversible Coma: Report of the Ad Hoc Committee of The Harvard Medical School to Examine the Definition of Brain Death, 204 J.A.M.A. 337 (1968).

20. Id.

21. Id.

22. Refinements in Criteria for the Determination of Death: An Appraisal, A Report of The Task Force on Death and Dying of The Institute of Safety, Ethics and the Life Sciences, 221 J.A.M.A. 50 (1972).

23. WASH. POST, April 22, 1981, at A27, col. 2.

24. 12 UNIF. LAWS ANN. 1 (1988 Supp.).

See Capron & Kass, A Statutory Definition of The Standards for Determining Human Death: An Appraisal and A Proposal, 121 U. PA. L. REV. 87 (1972).

25. ALA. CODE §22-31-1(b) (1975); NEV. REV. STAT. §451.007 (1979); W. VA. CODE §§16-10-1 to 16-10-3 (1980); WYO. STAT. §35-19-101 (1979).

See Comment, Medical-Legal Agreements on Brain Death: An Assessment of the Uniform Determination of Death Act, 8 J. CONTEMP. L. 97 (1982).

26. President's Commission for the Study of Ethical Problems in Medicine and Biomedical and Behavioral Research, DEFINING DEATH: MEDICAL, LEGAL AND ETHICAL ISSUES IN THE DETERMINATION OF DEATH 9, 10, 172, 173 (1981).

27. 12 UNIF. L. A. §1 (1985) Supp.).

28. ARK. STAT. ANN. §20-17-101 (1987); CAL. HEALTH & SAFETY CODE (West's Supp. 1988); COLO. REV. STAT. §12-36-136 (1985); DEL. CODE ANN. tit. 24, § 1760 (1987); D.C. CODE ANN. §6-2401 (Supp. 1988); GA. CODE ANN. §31-10-16 (1985); IDAHO CODE § 54-1819 (Supp. 1987); IND. CODE ANN. § 1-1-4-3 (Burns 1988); KAN. STAT. ANN. §§ 77-204 to 77-206 (1984); ME. REV. STAT. ANN. tit. 22, §§ 2811 to 2813 (Supp. 1988); MD. HEALTH–GEN. CODE ANN. § 5-202 (Supp. 1987); MISS. CODE ANN. §§41-36-1, 41-36-3 (1972); MO. ANN. STAT. § 194.005 (Vernon 1983); MONT. CODE ANN. § 50-22-101 (1987); NEV. REV. STAT. § 451.007 (1986); N.H. REV. STAT. ANN. §§141-D:1 to 141-D:2 (Supp. 1987); OHIO REV. CODE ANN. § 2108.30 (Page 1987); OKLA. STAT. ANN. tit. 63, §§ 3121 to 3123 (West Supp. 1988); OR. REV. STAT. § 432.300 (1987); PA. STAT. ANN. tit. 35, §§ 10201 to 10203 (Purdon's Supp. 1988); R.I. GEN. LAWS § 23-4-16 (1956); TENN. CODE ANN. § 68-3-501 (1987); S.C. CODE ANN. §§ 44-43-450, 44-43-460 (1976); VT. STAT. ANN. tit. 18, § 5218 (1987) and WYO. STAT. §§ 35-19-101 to 35-19-103 (1988).

29. Swafford v. State, _____ Ind. _____, 421 N.E. 2d 596, 602 (1981); *In re* Bowman, 94 Wash. 2d 407, 421, 617 P. 2d 731, 738 (1980).

30. Joynt, A New Look at Death, 252 J.A.M.A. 680, 681 (1984).

31. See generally, Abram, The Need for Uniform Law on The Determination of Death, 27 N.Y. LAW SCHOOL L. REV. 1187 (1981); J. FEINBERG, OFFENSE TO OTHERS (1984).

32. Smith, Legal Recognition of Neocortical Death, 71 CORNELL L. REV. 850 (1986).

33. Id. at 851.

34. Id. at 888.

35. Id.

36. President's Commission for the Study of Ethical Problems in Medicine and Biomedical and Behavioral Research, DECIDING TO FOREGO LIFE–SUSTAINING TREATMENT: ETHICAL, MEDICAL, AND LEGAL ISSUES IN TREATMENT DECISIONS 139 (1983) (hereinafter cited as President's Commission).

See generally, Kutner, Euthanasia: Due Process for Death with Dignity: The Living Will, 54 IND. L. J. 201 (1979).

37. President's Commission at 140.

38. Id.

One jurisdiction, the New Jersey Supreme Court, held *In re Conroy,* 98 N.J. 321, 351, 486 A. 2d 1209, 1224 (1985) that declining life sustaining medical treatment should not be viewed as an attempt to commit suicide.

39. ALA. CODE §§22-8A-1 to -10 (1984); ARIZ. REV. STAT. ANN. §§36-3201 to -3210 (1986); ARK. STAT. ANN. §82-3801 to -3804 (Supp. 1985); CAL. HEALTH & SAFETY CODE §§7185–7195 (West Supp. 1985); COLO. REV. STAT. §§15-18-101 to -113 (Supp. 1986); 1985 CONN. ACTS 85-606 (Reg. Sess.); DEL. CODE ANN. tit. 16, §§2501–2508 (1983); D.C. CODE ANN. §6-2421 to -2430 (Supp. 1986); FLA. STAT. §765.01–.15 (1986); GA. CODE ANN. §§31-32-1 to -12 (1985 & Supp. 1986); IDAHO CODE §§39-4501 to -4508 (1985 & Supp. 1986); ILL. ANN. STAT. ch. 110½, para. 701–710 (Smith-Hurd Supp. 1986); IND. CODE ANN. §§16-8-11-1 to -21 (Burns Supp. 1986); IOWA CODE ANN. §§144A.1 to .11 (West Supp. 1986); KAN. STAT. ANN. §65-28-101 to -109 (1980); LA. REV. STAT. ANN. §40:1299.58.1 to .10 (West Supp. 1986); ME. REV. STAT. ANN. tit. 22, §§2921 to 2931 (Supp. 1986); MD. HEALTH GEN. CODE ANN. §§5 -601 to -614 (Supp. 1986); MISS. CODE ANN. §§41-41-101 to -121 (Supp. 1985); MO. ANN. STAT. §§459.010 to .055 (Vernon Supp. 1986); MONT. CODE ANN. §§50-9-101 to -111 (1985); NEV. REV. STAT. §§449.540 -690 (1986); N.H. REV. STAT. ANN. §§137-14:1 to -:16 (Supp. 1985); N.M. STAT. ANN. §§24-7-1 to -11 (1986); N.C. GEN. STAT. §§90-320 to -322 (1985); OKLA. STAT. ANN. tit. 63, §§3101 to 3111 (West Supp. 1987); OR. REV. STAT. §§97.050 to .090 (1985); TENN. CODE ANN. 32-11-101 to -110 (Supp. 1986); TEX. REV. CIV. STAT. ANN. art. 4590h (Vernon Supp. 1986); UTAH CODE ANN. §§75-2-1101 to -1118 (Supp. 1986); VT. STAT. ANN. tit. 18, §§5251 to 5262 (Supp. 1985); VA. CODE ANN. §§54-325.8:1 to :13 (Supp. 1986); WASH. REV. CODE ANN. §§70.122.010 to .905 (Supp. 1986); W. VA. CODE §§16-30-1 to -10 (1985); WIS. STAT. ANN. §§154.01 to .15 (West Supp. 1986); WYO. STAT. §§33-26-144 to -152 (Supp. 1986). See Gelfand, Living Will Statutes: The First Decade, 1987 Wisc. L. Rev. 737.

40. J. NOWAK, R. ROTUNDA, J. YOUNG, CONSTITUTIONAL LAW 765 (2d ed. 1983).

41. Id.

42. Twenty-one states and the District of Columbia have either natural death or death with dignity legislation: ALA. CODE §§22-8A-1 to 22-8A-10 (Supp. 1982); ARK. STAT. ANN. §§82-3801 to 82-3804 (Michie Supp. 1983); CAL. HEALTH & SAFETY CODE §§7185-95 (West Supp. 1983); DEL. CODE ANN. tit 16, §§2501-09 (1983); D.C. CODE ANN. §§6-2421 to 6-2430 (Michie Supp. 1983); LIFE–PROLONGING PROCEDURE ACT OF FLORIDA, ch. 84-58, 3 FLA. SESS. LAW SERV. 40 (West 1984); GA. CODE ANN. §§31-32-1 to 31-32-12 (Michie Supp. 1984); Idaho Code §§39-4501 to 39-4508 (Michie Supp. 1983); ILL. ANN. STAT. ch. 110½, §§701–710 (Smith-Hurd Supp. 1984–85); KAN. STAT. ANN. §§65-28, 101 to 65-28, 101 to 65-28, 109 (1980); Act. of Apr. 16, 1984, ch. 365, 1984 Miss. Law 98; NEV. REV. STAT. §§449.540 to 449.690 (1983); N.M. STAT. ANN. §§24-77-1 to 24-7-11 (1981); N.C. GEN. STAT. §§90-320 to 90-323 (1981); OR. REV. STAT. §§97.050 to 97.090 (1981); TEX. REV. CIV. STAT. ANN. art. 4590h (Vernon Supp. 1983); VT. STAT. ANN. tit. 18, §§5251–5262 (Supp. 1984); VA. CODE §§54-325.8:1 to 54-325.8:13

(Michie Supp. 1985); WASH. REV. CODE ANN. §§70.122.010 to 70.122.905 (West Supp. 1983–84); W. VA. CODE §§16-30-1 to 16-30-10 (Michie Supp. 1984); WIS. STAT. ANN. §§154.01 to 154.15 (Supp. 1985); WYO. STAT. §§33-26-144 to 33-26-152 (Michie Supp. 1984).

At pages 318–387 of the President's Commission (Report), may be found a verbatim reproduction of the state Natural Death Acts.

43. President's Commission at 141.

44. Id.

45. See CAL. HEALTH & SAFETY CODE §§7187(e), 7191(b) (Deering Supp. 1982).

In *Bartling v. Superior Court of Los Angeles County (Glendale Adventist Center)*, 163 Cal. App. 3d 186, 209 Cal. Rptr. 226 (1984), the court observed that even with a set of statutory guidelines as those found in the California Natural Death Act, such guidelines were "so cumbersome that it is unlikely that any but a small number of high educated and motivated patients will be able to effectuate their desires." 163 Ca. App. 3d at 194, n. 5, 209 Cal. Rptr. at 224, n. 5 (quoting *Barber v. Superior Court of Los Angeles County*, 147 Cal. App. 3d 1006 at 1015, 195 Cal. Rptr. 484 at 489 (1983).

46. President's Commission at 144.

47. Id.

48. Id.

49. Id.

50. See e.g., Natural Death Act, CAL. HEALTH & SAFETY CODE §7188 (West Supp. 1984); Natural Death Act, KAN. STAT. ANN. §§65-28, 102 (1980); Withholding or Withdrawal of Life Sustaining Procedures, NEV. REV. STAT. §499.590.610 (1983); Natural Death Act, WASH. REV. CODE ANN. §70.122.020 (Supp. 1985).

51. N.C. GEN. STAT. §90.322 (1981 & Supp. 1983).

52. VA. CODE §54-325.8:1 (Supp. 1985).

See generally, Comment, Proxy Decisionmaking for the Terminally Ill: The Virginia Approach, 70 VA. L. REV. 1269 (1984).

53. N.M. STAT. ANN. §24-7-4 (1981).

54. ARK. STAT. ANN. §82-3803 (Michie Supp. 1983).

55. President's Commission at 145, 146.

56. ALASKA STAT. §13.26.325 (1973); ARIZ. REV. STAT. ANN. §14-5501 (1975); ARK. STAT. ANN. §§58 to 501-511 (1971); CAL. ANN. CIV. CODE §§2400 to 2407 (Deering 1983); COLO. REV. STAT. §15-14-501 (Cum. Supp. 1982); DEL. CODE ANN. tit. 12, §§4901 to 4905 (Cum. Supp. 1982); FLA. STAT. §709.08 (Cum. Pocket Part 1983); GA. CODE ANN., §10-6-36 (1982); HAWAII REV. STAT., §560:5-501 (Supp. 1981); IDAHO CODE §§15-5-501 to 502 (1982); IND. CODE §30-2-1.5-1 (1981); IOWA CODE ANN., §633.705 (West 1983); KAN. STAT. ANN., §§58-610 to 617 (Cum. Supp. 1981); KY. REV. STAT. ANN., §386.093 (Baldwin 1982); *Succession of McCrocklin*, 242 La. 404, 137 So. 2d 74 (1962); ME. REV. STAT. ANN., tit. 18-A, §5-501 (1964); MD. EST. & TRUSTS CODE ANN. §13-601 (1974); MASS. GEN. LAWS ANN., ch. 201B, §§1 to 7 (West 1981); MICH. STAT. ANN. §27.5495 (Callagan 1980); MINN. STAT. §524.5-501 (West 1976); MONT. CODE ANN. §§75-5-501 to 502 (1981); NEB. REV. STAT. §30-2662 (1979); N.J. STAT. ANN. §§46:2B-8 (West Cum.

Supp. 1982–83); N.M. STAT. ANN. §45-5-501 (1978); N.Y. GEN. OBLIG. LAW §5-1601 (McKinney 1978); N.C. GEN. STAT. §47-115.1 (Cum. Supp. 1981); N.D. CENT. CODE §30.1-30-01 (1976); OHIO REV. CODE ANN., §1337.09 (Page 1979); OKLA. STAT. ANN. tit. 58, §§1051 to 1062 (West 1983); ORE. REV. STAT. §126.407 (1981); 20 PA. CONS. STAT. ANN. §5601 (Purdon 1976); S.C. CODE ANN., §32-13-10 (Cum. Supp. 1982); S.D. CODIFIED LAWS ANN. §§59-7-2.1 to 59-7-2.4 (1978); TENN. CODE ANN. §66-5-105 (1982); TEX. REV. CIV. STAT. ANN. art. 36A (Vernon 1980); UTAH CODE ANN. §75-5-501 (1978); VT. STAT. ANN. tit. 14, §3051 (1982); VA. CODE §§11-9.1 through 11-9.2 (1978); WASH. REV. CODE §11.94.010 (1982); W. VA. CODE §27-11-6 (1982); WIS. STAT. ANN. §243.07 (West 1982); WYO. STAT., §34-9-101 to 110 (1977).

At pages 393–437 of the President's Commission (Report), may be found verbatim reproductions of the Durable Power of Attorney statutes found in the Report of the Commission.

See generally, Martyn & Jacobs, Legislating Advance Directives for the Terminally Ill: The Living Will and Durable Power of Attorney, 63 NEB. L. REV. 779 (1984).

57. President's Commission at 147.

58. Id.

59. Id. at 146.

60. Id. at 147.

61. Id.

62. Unif. Rights of the Terminally Ill Act, 9A UNIF. L. ANN. §§1–18 (Supp. Pamph. 1987).

63. Defined as "any medical procedure or intervention that, when administered to a qualified patient, will serve only to prolong the process of dying." Sec. 1(4).

64. Defined as "an incurable or irreversible condition that, without the administration of life-sustaining treatment, will, in the opinion of the attending physician, result in death within a relatively short time." Sec. 1(9).

65. See Marzen, The Uniform Rights of The Terminally Ill Act: A Critical Analysism, 1 ISSUES LAW & MED. 441 (May 1986).

66. Humane and Dignified Death Initiative, Sec. 1(a) proposed as amendment to Art. 1 of the Calif. Const.

See also, Bond, Hemlock Society Forms New Organization to Push Assisted Suicide Initiative, *National Right to Life News,* Dec. 18, 1986, at 1, col. 1; Bishop, Backers Fail to get Lethal Injection Bid on California Ballot, N.Y. Times, May 18, 1988, at 23, col. 1.

67. §7188, Humane and Dignified Death Act.

The hope is that the 500,000 signatures necessary to place the issue on referendum will be achieved by November, 1988. Derek Humphrey, executive director of the Hemlock Society of California, is rather confident the necessary signatures supporting the initiative will be obtained because " . . . the national polls show that 60 percent of the public supports suicide assistance for terminally ill patients and another 12 percent is undecided on the issue." Price, Pro-suicide activists call for a Right to Assist, WASH. TIMES, Mar. 13, 1987, at 6A, col. 2.

68. Id. at §7188.5.

69. Id. at §7189(a).

70. Id. at §7189(b), §7195.

71. Id. at §7191(c).

72. Id. at §7192.

73. Id. at §2443.

74. Id.

75. See generally, Kuhse, The Case for Active Voluntary Euthanasia, 14 LAW, MED. & HEALTH CARE 145 (Sept. 1986); Engelhardt & Malloy, Suicide and Assisting Suicide: A Critique of Legal Sanctions, 36 SO. W. L.J. 1003 (1982).

76. Morrison, Death: Process or Event?, 173 SCIENCE 694, 695 (Aug. 20, 1971).

77. Id.

Chapter IV

EUTHANSIA

THE RIGHT TO A GOOD DEATH

Since theology and ethics are logically independent, there is no need, within the context of moral arguments, to reply to theological objections or become captives of them.[1] Yet, traditional moral attitudes regarding euthanasia are affected profoundly by theological ideas—and three in particular: that God, alone, has total dominion and control over all human life; death is a form of punishment and to kill innocent life places one's soul in jeopardy of eternal damnation. These points have—in one form or other—been discussed previously.[2] It is well to re-state them here as a prefatory acknowledgment to this chapter of the book and to underscore, again, the foundation for past reference to euthanasia.

If a "right to die" is but merely a right to the inevitable,[3] the proper question to be raised is why the claim to the inevitable? And the answer lies—as has been seen—in a recognition of the vast technologics of medical science that make life almost endless.[4] Advanced medical devices that make respiration, cardiac massage, uterine curettage, intravenous feeding and a limitless availability of antibiotics not only forestall death but introduce untold confusion and lack of agreement in determining when in fact it occurs.[5]

Because a "good" death is now quite improbable for most, it is understandable that a majority of individuals, when asked the manner in which death would be preferable, reply that a death without warning (as with an accident) is their choice. The most common fear remains that of dying under protracted circumstances in a hospital, the *victim* of modern technological processes. Thus, according to present levels of conception, or misconception as the case may be, "the only way left for a person to die in euthanasia is to be killed somehow."[6]

For the bioethicist, the right to die with dignity is grounded in one basic principle: avoid human distress.[7] The right, itself, may be recognized as having three ethical parts that conduce to the whole: a right to have full information provided one by his physician regarding his medical problem—its origin and prognosis—in order that he may, in turn, give an informed consent to treatment or non-treatment as the case may be; a right to both "human company and care" that includes not only relief from pain, but the maintenance of a treating environment free of noxious stimuli; and, finally, a right to die unmolested by meddlesome procedures that would include a right to refuse this and other forms of treatment.[8] This composite interest in a right to die continues to be obscured and generally frustrated by the present use of the term, "euthanasia," in all its stated and more subtle definitional and practical applications.

Euthanasia, as a term, concept, or attitude has been used under various and confusing circumstances to denote "any good death," "any assistance in helping dying patients in their dying (including the cessation of treatments)", and "only acting directly to kill the dying patient."[9] The intriguing fact emerging from any study of euthanasia, then, will be that it can mean "any good death" as well as a "morally outrageous death."[10]

Active euthanasia, then, involves killing while passive euthanasia does not; one is not acceptable, the other is being tolerated and accepted more and more. But, query: how can letting die be in some way preferable— from a moral standpoint—than helping die? If all other morally relevant factors—intention, motivation, outcome—are the same, why should there be a difference? In truth, the difference between killing and letting die has no moral significance.

> In active euthanasia, the doctor initiates a course of events that lead to the patient's death.... In letting die, the agent stands back and lets nature take her sometimes cruel course.... [11]

The traditional argument against adoption or acceptance of euthanasia is that a rational patient simply does not and cannot choose euthanasia.[12] If this were so, it would have to be maintained further that no autonomous and rational decision could ever be made by a patient to refuse a modality of treatment that was life sustaining.[13] Yet, this is not what the vast majority of active euthanasia opponents assert. Rather, they maintain that a patient can in fact make a rational choice to follow passive euthanasia—but not active euthanasia.[14] The inconsistency is obvious. The crucial question that begs answering is: Whether a patient "can rationally choose an earlier death over a later one...."[15] Accordingly, it is submitted that if one can make a rational choice to follow passive euthanasia, then he must also be entitled to make a rational choice to follow active euthanasia[17] or, as termed in this article, "enlightened self-determination."[17]

BENEFICENT EUTHANASIA

Beneficent euthanasia is defined simply as the painless inducement of a quick death.[18] The most common paradigm of it would include cases where an individual suffers from an irreversible condition such as disseminated carcinoma metastasis, has excruciating and indurable pain, is beyond reasonable medical doubt that death is imminent, is told of his condition and requests some means of "easy death" and aside from a desire to help such an individual, no other relevant conditions exist.[19]

The crux of the argument for beneficent euthanasia is found in what is termed a societal obligation "to treat members kindly"[20] consistent with a principle of beneficence.[21] Suffering should at all times be minimized and kindly treatment maximized.[22] This position should be able to be advocated without fear of it being viewed in reality as another Nazi-type plan for extermination.[23] The fear that the use of euthanasia—however qualified—runs the risk of destroying the social fabric of society is unfounded.[24] Beneficent euthanasia's utilization is consistent totally with the basic human need for dignity or self-respect. It should not be viewed as a punishment, but rather simply as a matter of meeting this basic need and—at the same time—executing the societal obligation or collective responsibility of treating all members of society kindly or with compassion.[25]

Perhaps at the heart of any discussion of euthanasia is whether such life-ending acts are cruel in and of themselves[26] and morally justified. As important, is a consideration of whether in point of fact the act of euthanasia is administered to a *person.*[27] For one to be recognized as a person, it is commonly regarded as necessary for him to have rational awareness.[28] Query: is a "betubed, sedated, aerated, glucosed, mechanically manipulated" individual one capable of being considered rationally aware?[29] Arguably, one simply is not a person under these conditions[30] and the individual who acts deliberately and with set purpose to relieve such suffering of an incurably ill and extremely debilitated individual should not be recognized as having committed an act of murder.[31] But, for this conclusion to have merit, some type of set criteria or characteristics for personhood must be acknowledged as either correct or acceptable,[32] or an incontrovertible definition of it agreed upon.[33] An analysis of the requisites of personhood and their value as a construct for critical decision making has been previously analyzed.[34] Suffice it to note only by way of re-emphasis that these various criteria have yet to achieve the mark of incontrovertibility. Yet, there is very wide agreement that when there is no "relational potential" or a capacity for love and engaging in interpersonal relations—owing to an absence of cerebral functioning—there can be no recognition of personhood.[35]

BLURRED DEFINITIONS
AND A POSITED CLARIFICATION

A good number of physicians and moral theologians use "euthanasia" only in connection with active euthanasia, preferring as such to refer to "passive euthanasia" as "the right to death with dignity."[36] The reality of the present situation is that many of the old, chronically ill, debilitated or mentally impaired are *allowed* to die by withholding the agressive medical treatment and available care as do young, mentally normal patients.[37]

Since little if any substance depends upon what label is attached to these present actions under consideration, the debate about the distinctions becomes pointless.[38] Indeed, because of the blurring of distinctions between active and passive euthanasia, there is really no distinct difference between the two.[39]

> If death is intentionally caused by doing something or withholding something there is no morally significant distinction to be drawn between an active means to death and a passive means to death. Both are alike or intended means to death; and both the intention and the result are the same—the death of the patient. If one simply withholds treatment, it may take the patient longer to die, and he may suffer more than he would if more direct action were taken and a lethal injection given.[40]

In an effort to establish clarity of analysis, it has been suggested to re-define euthanasia as either the putting to death or the failure to prevent death in cases of terminal illness or injury.[41] The motives behind such an act would be to either relieve comatoseness, the effects of permanent suffering, anxiety or perhaps a perceived sense of burdensomeness.[42] Thus, as newly clarified, at least one other person would be seen as causing or helping to cause the death of a competent individual who desires death; or, in the case of an incompetent, makes a substituted decision regarded as in the individual's best interests to either cause death directly or to withdraw some mechanism or process that sustains life.[43]

In its Declaration of Venice of October, 1983, the World Medical Assembly concluded that the best interests of the patient should be the operative standard under which health care matters are decided upon.[44] Although this would appear to be a principle grounded in common sense and pre-eminently reasonable as well, there are a number of growing situations or cases where the medical profession operates counter to the best interests of many of its patients. Letting die, to be more specific, often involves a course of *inaction* that directly conflicts with the best interests of a patient. An illustrative case dramatizes this vividly.

> A woman is dying of terminal cancer of the throat. She is no longer able to take food and fluids by mouth and is suffering considerable distress. She would be able to live for a few more weeks if medical feeding by way of a nasogastric tube were continued. However, the woman does not want the extra two or three weeks of life because life has become a burden which she no longer wishes to bear. She asks the doctor to help her die. The doctor agrees to discontinue medical feeding, removes the nasogastric tube, and the woman dies a few days later.[45]

Death was obviously in the best interests of this woman. The *method*, however, for allowing its occurrence was not. If a lethal injection had been given, a quick and painless death would have resulted. Rather, after having the nasogastric tube removed, she lingered a few days—dying ultimately of dehydration and starvation.[46] Was it in this patient's "best interests" to be starved to death? Did society in some manner triumph because this individual was forced to suffer an undignified ending but avoided being "killed" mercifully?[47]

The sad, but very real, fact is that a swift and painless death is not always the result that follows from cessation of life-sustaining treatment.[48] For, the patient whose kidneys have failed, and dialysis or transplant surgery is not pursued, while generally remaining conscious will experience normally one or all of the following: nausea and vomiting, an inability to concentrate and—eventually—convulsions.[49] What type of justification can be given for utilizing a method of treatment involving more suffering, instead of loss, as being in an individual's best interests?

ACTS OF TREATMENT V. OMISSIONS OF TREATMENT

In classical Greece, medicine was given three roles: to alleviate the sufferings of the sick; lessen the violence of diseases that afflicted them and "refusing to treat those who are overmastered by their diseases, realizing that in such cases medicine was powerless."[50] Indeed, the most common duty of all Greco-Roman physicians was "to help, or least to do no harm."[51] It was a pure matter of discretion when a hopeless case was taken by a physician.[52] This prevailing sentiment of physicians in this period of civilization found strong precedent in Egyptian and Assyro-Babylonian medicine.[53] As a medical sentiment, in fact, it continued in vitality throughout the Middle Ages.[54] It is commonly thought that Francis Bacon, writing in his, *De augmentis scientiarium,* in the late 16th and early 17th centuries, advanced the conclusion that medicine should seek to prolong life and expand longevity, and the notion has grown in an exaggerated and misdirected manner since that time.[55]

So it is seen, then, that while a physician's so-called duty to prolong life *qua* life has no classical roots, the idea of "respect for life" does have a rich tradition of observance.[56] But, to be remembered, is the fact that even though physicians would not actively seek to terminate a life either by abortion or euthanasia, they were also *not* required to actively prolong life, itself.[57] While, with the rise of Christianity, abortion, suicide and euthanasia became sins, still the prolongation of life never did "become either a virtue or a duty."[58]

Morality of Actions

Pope John Paul II approved the "Declaration of Euthanasia" adopted by the Sacred Congregation for the Doctrine of Faith on May 5, 1980, and in so doing advanced broad principles of humanistic care and treatment for the dying.[59] Acknowledging that one may seek to utilize advanced medical techniques of an experimental and high-risk nature in order to combat an illness, the Declaration allows for the interruption of these processes when they render unsatisfactory results.[60] But before actions of this nature are allowed, the patient's "reasonable wishes" and those of his family, together with the advice of the attending physicians, must be considered.[61] Deferring to the physicians expertise in matters of this nature, the Declaration allows that they "may in particular judge that the investment in instruments and personnel is *disproportionate to the results foreseen.*"[62] And that, further, they may conclude that, "the techniques applied impose on the patient strain or suffering *out of proportion* with the benefits which he or she may gain from such techniques."[63] What is seen here is a clear and unequivocable example of a cost vs. benefit analysis which has been submitted is a proper standard of evaluation.

One may, of course, consistent with the Declaration, "make do with the normal means that medicine can offer."[64] Thus, if such a course is followed, "one cannot impose on anyone the obligation to have recourse to a technique which is already in use but which *carries a risk or is burdensome.*"[65] A refusal of this type is not in any way to be regarded as an act equivalent to suicide — but rather an acceptance of a human condition — a desire to avoid the use of a modality of treatment "disproportionate to the results" or a wish to prevent excessive financial drains on the patient's family "or the community."[66] Again, the element of economic feasibility of treatment is set forth as a proper vector of force in ultimate decision making. The need to ration scarce medical resources so that they may be expended on those who have a real possibility of recovery is also impliedly recognized in the Declaration.[67]

The Declaration concluded that, "When inevitable death is imminent in spite of the means used, it is permitted in conscience to take the decision to refuse forms of treatment that would only secure a precarious and burdensome prolongation of life, so long as the normal care due to the sick person in similar cases is not interrupted."[68]

Ordinary v. Extraordinary Treatment

The principles of ordinary versus extraordinary life-sustaining processes or treatments are very relative — not only as to time and locale, but also in their application to specific cases. In essence, these concepts serve as basic value judgments that aid in reaching a determination whether a given modality of treatment presents an undue hardship on the at-risk patient or whether it provides hope for a direct benefit. Thus, if too great a hardship would be imposed on the patient by following a particular medical or surgical course of treatment and no reasonable *hope of benefit* was to be derived therefrom, such actions would be viewed properly as extraordinary and not obligatory.[69] In practice, many physicians choose to equate "ordinary" with "usual," and "extraordinary" with "unusual" or "heroic" medical practice.[70] Once it has been decided to withhold "heroics," no rational process has been developed that facilitates decision making regarding what treatment should be pursued and what withheld. Indeed, sometimes half-treatments are initiated thereby allowing, for example, intravenous feeding but at a rate that will result in dehydration over time.[71] Such a gesture maintains the vital symbol of feeding that does not sustain the life of the patient over an extended period of time.[72] Although somewhat deceiving, it nonetheless serves as a type of artificial compromise for those wishing to respect the symbol yet at the same time act in accordance with patient's needs and, often, his present or previously expressed wishes.[73]

Determining whether medical or surgical treatment is either ordinary or extraordinary may be regarded as a quality of life statement. And, in reaching this statement, knowingly or unknowingly, the decision makers involved (legal, medical, ethical) utilize a substituted judgment to conclude whether—in and under similar circumstances to that which the patient *in extremis* exists—they would or would not wish to survive in such a physical and mental state. Obviously, decisions of this moment are made within a varied and yet complex vortex of highly charred emotions.[74]

If love be recognized as the binding force of life, it may be submitted that man should endeavor to seek to maximize a response to life in whatever assorted conditions or states he finds himself existing and, at the same time, minimize suffering and maximize the social good or utility of life.[75] Thus, very simply stated, if an act when undertaken would cause more harm than good to or for the at-risk individual in question *and* to those associated closely with him, the act could be considered an unloving one. The central point to be understood is that, in cases of this nature, a basic cost/benefit analysis is almost always undertaken—be it on a conscious or unconscious level.[76]

On a case-by-case, or situational basis with the standard of reasonableness as the lynch-pin—as opposed to an unyielding *a priori* ethic—health care providers should balance the gravity of the harm caused by extraordinary care, against the utility of the good that will result from such extraordinary actions. As such, the decision makers should be ever mindful of the ethical imperative to minimize human suffering at all levels when making ultimate decisions.[77] In reality, it is submitted that this mandated balancing test validates a cost/benefit analysis.[78] It is only after, however, recognizing that all life is sanctified by creation, and is not only qualitative to the individual at peril as well as to mankind in general, that inquiry may proceed to be made into whether the medically handicapped individual possesses a sustained ability to enjoy and fulfill loving, interpersonal relationships with others; and whether the present or contemplated course of medical or surgical treatment maximizes that potential utility of life—assuming it exists—or, contrariwise minimizes present suffering.[79]

Measures of an extraordinary nature undertaken for the specific purpose of prolonging a life of suffering should be recognized as not only unjust to the individual in distress but as an act of effrontery to the societal standard of decency and humanity.[80] The physician's primary responsibility is to relieve suffering when it occurs—not to seek the survival of a patient at all costs. Indeed, an overly aggressive modality of treatment for a terminally ill patient—regardless of age—should be recognized as a defilement of the very doctrine of *primum non nocere.* If therapy would be futile and to no end other than mere survival, it should not be administered.[81] Thus, the artificial feeding of a terminally ill patient in irreversible coma should be regarded as a *treatment* decision and not mandated except when benefits clearly outweigh burdens.[82]

Moralists suggest that three commonly accepted principles are at the center of the individual's—and not his relatives or the medical profession—responsibility to preserve his life:

> *Per se* he is obliged to use the ordinary means of preserving his life. *Per se* he is not obliged to use extraordinary means, though the use of such means is permissible and generally commendable. *Per accidens,* however, he is obliged to use even extraordinary means, if the preservation of his life is required for some greater good such as his own spiritual welfare or the common good.[83]

Application of the Principle of Double Effect, although recognized as an exception to these three controlling principles, is not extended to those cases regarded as *morally impossible;* thus the use of extraordinary means is not included within the principle, itself.[84]

The investment of economic and social resources in prolonging one's life, where such actions constitute an inordinate drain on familial and societal resources and achieve little more than merely extending the dying process, are not mandated morally under the ordinary-extraordinary principle.[85] Indeed, the very concept of ordinary means for preserving life has been defined as, " . . . all medicines, treatments, and operations, which offer a reasonable hope of benefit for the patient and which can be obtained and used without excessive expense, pain or other inconvenience."[86] Contraiwise, extraordinary or optional means of treatment are taken to be all those medicines, treatments or surgeries that are incapable of being administered without excessive outlays of money or other inconveniences and—if in fact followed—would offer no reasonable hope of recovery or positive benefit.[87] The likelihood of success in undertaking the treatment is a valid consideration.[88] Accordingly, if for example a class of newborns for whom treatment would be so prohibitively costly and so unlikely of success could be identified, treatment would be excused.[89]

A number of relative factors must be weighed in deciding whether to excuse a modality of treatment. As noted, the successfulness of the proposed treatment is a major factor for consideration; and, of course, there are degrees of success. While it is one matter to administer oxygen in order to alleviate a medical crisis for a patient, it is another matter to use that same oxygen to merely prolong a life for which recovery is negligible. Degrees of hope are a second factor to be evaluated when it concerns complete recovery. Thus, while in one case oxygen is administered in order to end a patient's bout with pneumonia and may and usually does offer a very high hope of complete recovery, in other cases the patient's physical condition may be so fragile that there is but an equally fragile hope of recovery from the medical crisis. The degrees of difficulty in obtaining and using ordinary means comprise the third set of factors; for some means are easy to obtain and use and are inexpensive and others are much more difficult to obtain and to use.[90]

Intravenous feeding problems present a unique paradigm for study of the ordinary-extraordinary conundrum. One case study is illustrative:

> A cancer patient is in extreme pain and his system has gradually established what physicians call 'toleration' of any drug, so that even increased doses give only brief respites from the ever-recurring pain. The attending physician knows that the disease is incurable and that the person is slowly dying, but because of a good heart, it is possible that the agony will continue for several weeks. The physician then remembers that there is one thing he can do to end the suffering. He can cut off intravenous feeding and the patient will surely die. He does this and before the next day the patient is dead.
>
> The case involves the principle that an ordinary means of prolonging life and an extraordinary means are relative to the patient's physical condition. Intravenous feeding is an artificial means of prolonging life and therefore one may be more liberal in application of principle. Since this cancer patient is beyond all hope of recovery and suffering extreme pain, intravenous feeding should be considered an extraordi-

nary means of prolonging life. The physician was justified in stopping the intravenous feeding. . . . [91]

Further subtleties and ambiguities in the taxonomy of ordinary versus extraordinary care are seen dramatically in three landmark case opinions. In the case of *In re Dinnerstein* the Court observed that its task was to discern the rather slight "distinction between those situations in which the withholding of extraordinary measures may be viewed as allowing the disease to take its natural course and those in which the same actions may be deemed to have been the cause of death."[92] The Court in *Superintendent of Belchertown State School v. Saikewicz* stated that no extraordinary means of prolonging life should be pursued when there is no hope that the patient will recover. "Recovery should not be defined simply as the ability to remain alive, it should mean life without intolerable suffering."[93] Finally, in *In re Quinlan,* the Court opined, "One would have to think that the use of the same respirator or life support could be considered 'ordinary' in the context of the possibly curable patient but 'extraordinary' in the context of the forced sustaining by cardio-respiratory processes of an *irreversibly doomed patient.* "[94]

Circularity in Terminology

It has been suggested that both the terms, ordinary and extraordinary medical treatment, are "incurably circular until filled with concrete or descriptive meaning,"[95] and that—furthermore—this language be abandoned in favor of a classification that merely recognizes "treatment medically indicated" for a non-dying or salvageable, which would thus be expected to be helpful, and "curative treatment not indicated (for the dying)."[96] Of course, the central weakness of this posture is that no objective criteria or concreteness is set forth with this classification itself that would enable a decision maker to act unerringly. No guiding or unyielding *a priori* standard is proferred—only a standard of situational reasonableness tied to the facts of each case. Perhaps, however, within this "weakness" is to be found the very strength of the suggestion: a straight recognition that no definitive position can be taken.

Another suggestion has been to ban the artificial distinctions between ordinary/extraordinary treatment focus—instead—on whether, in a given case, medical treatment is "morally imperative" or merely "elective."[97] For a competent patient, a refusal of treatment would be accepted when he could present reasons relevant to this declining physical or mental health or to familial, social, economic or religious concerns, that were valid to him and him alone.[98] The incompetent patient is faced with the knowing reality that he is unable to make reasonable choices. Thus, the decision maker in this setting—spouse, parent, child, next of kin, guardian or physician—may refuse treatment on morally acceptable grounds when such an action would seem "within the realm of reason to reasonable people."[99]

The question remains: What is the test of reasonableness?

> A reasonable person would find a refusal unreasonable (and thus treatment morally required) if the treatment is useful in treating a patient's condition (though not necessarily life-saving) and at the same time does not give use to any significant patient-centered objections based on physical or mental burden; familial, social, or economic concern; or religious belief.[100]

Both of these new classifications regarding ordinary/extraordinary treatment are inescapably tied to a standard or qualitative living—perceived as such by the at-risk patient, his family or supportive network or health care decision maker. Does this mean that all ultimate decisions regarding treatment or nontreatment are essentially cost-benefit ones? The feasibility of structuring a framework for principled decision making or, for that matter, a construct to aid in decision of this nature will be explored in Chapter VI.

Suffice it to suggest at this juncture that ideally the concepts of ordinary and extraordinary means of treatment should be disregarded totally not only because of their imprecise terms of definition and application but also because they tend to support paternalism.[101] While the standards of customary medical practice determine what ought to be done, both the disease entity together with the medical technologies needed to treat it displace the patient as the focus of concern. Indeed, the patient-person becomes subordinated totally to the patient-disease-bearer.[102] What is demanded, then, is a simple recognition that no form of treatment is either obligatory or optional. Rather, everything depends upon the condition of the patient.[103] Thus,

> The only adequate grounds or standards can be found in the ratio of benefits and burdens of the treatment to the patient. But a competent patient should make his or her own assessment, while a proxy must make it for an incompetent patient, using that patient's previously expressed wishes or values when they can be determined.[104]

THE PRINCIPLE OF DOUBLE EFFECT

The principles of Indirect or Double Effect, one of the basic principles of Catholic medical ethics,[105] and one also intuited by many others not necessarily members of the Roman Church, is best understood by an understanding—or often times but a vague feeling—that the administration of a potentially lethal narcotic that would relieve the intractable pain of a cancer patient is in some way different—morally—from a knowing act that would murder the same patient, justifying it on the grounds of acting mercifully.[106] Stated otherwise,

> The principle is intended to provide a halfway ground between a straightforward utilitarianism, which would simply consider the relative weights of the good and bad consequences of an action in order to make a moral judgment of it, and a variety of sterner moral positions, which would either deny the moral relevance of consequences to actions altogether or would judge immoral any action with bad consequences, no matter what other good consequences it had.[107]

The net result of recognizing and applying the Principle of Double Effect is that certain actions *indirectly* producing certain evil consequences are justified—so long as four conditions are met: the action undertaken, independent of its effect, must not itself be inherently held to be morally evil; the evil effect must not be utilized as a means to produce the good effect; the evil effect is merely tolerated and not sincerely intended and, finally, regardless of its evil consequences, there is a proportionate reason for undertaking the action.[108] Utilization of this principle provides the justification, for example, of removing a cancerous fetus-bearing uterus and the administration of pain-relieving narcotics that may—in turn—produce respiratory depression.[109] The Principle's legitimacy has been attacked, alternatively, because it leads to discriminations that are wrongful by excusing acts (or thought to be killings, by some) it should not and forbidding other such acts it should allow.[110]

A principle of such ambivalence is open—obviously—to these and other logical deficiencies. But, it has been suggested that validation is recognized because of its "psychological validity."[111] A use-hypothetical attempts to bring into focus this point. Faced with a patient's intolerable pain and his pleas for relief that cannot be mitigated by lesser doses of non-lethal drugs, a physician chooses to administer a dose of an analgesic that will likely cause death. A crucial contrast is then undertaken between the attitude and the manner that the motive for relieving pain engenders compared with attitudes and manner pursued when a premeditated act to kill is pursued.[112]

> If the purpose explicitly were to kill, would there not be profound difference in the very way one would grasp the syringe, the look in the eye, the words that might be spoken or withheld, those subtle admixtures of fear and hope that haunt the death-bed scene? And would not the consequences of the difference be compounded almost geometrically at least for the physician as he killed one such patient after another? And what of the repercussions of the difference on the nurses and hospital attendants? How long would the quality and attitude of mercy survive death-intending conduct? The line between the civilized and savage in men is fine enough without jeopardizing it by euthanasia. History teaches the line is maintainable under the principle of double effect; it might well not be under a regime of direct intentional killing.[113]

Whether the lessons of history substantiate the alleged "psychological validity" of the principle and establish that it is efficacious—that it merits its ready use and retention seem dubious, at best. Rather than continue to enshrine an awkward concept, it should be replaced by the relatively simple and enduring standard of what is, under a given set of facts, *reasonable*. Guided or supported by the principle of *triage* and a consideration of what actions are in the best interests of the at-risk patient, a cost/benefit analysis should be undertaken in order to decide whether one modality of treatment or non-treatment should be pursued.[114] Thus, reasonable, humane and cost-effective actions should be both the procedure utilized and the goal sought here.

The intensive care unit found within the average hospital in the United States not only seeks to treat and to return patients suffering from serious injuries or acute diseases to their original working or stabilized environments but also to serve as a sophisticated, state-of-the-art hospice.[115] Even when there is no hope of recovery, studies have shown that approximately nineteen percent of patients in ICU's are nonetheless admitted and stay.[116] It would seem to be a reasonable and sensible idea for at-risk patients to decide not to be treated in an intensive care unit; this choice not being made necessarily with the idea of dying sooner, but rather with the view in mind that access to family and friends will be more easily facilitated as well as family and social and economic resources conserved.[117]

Choices of this nature should not be confused or tied to the Principle of Double Effect. Rather, when tragic choices are simply not between different chances of survival with different treatments but only between extending the process of suffering and death or shortening it, the principle has little pertinence or significance.[118]

> Patients may very well sensibly decide to forego treatment or ICU care so that they may in fact finally die and end their travail. They may directly will their deaths and thus within one strict interpretation of moral theory, passively commit suicide.[119]

Physicians in England are not allowed to initiate any actions that have, as their primary purpose, to cause a patient's death.[120] Accordingly, under the Suicide Act of 1961, if a physician were to endeavor to facilitate the request of a terminally ill patient for assistance in terminating his life, he would subject himself to criminal prosecution.[121] A physician is also, under this legislation, not allowed to honor suggestions from the family of a gravely ill patient to end the life of such a patient.[122] Yet, since one of the basic commitments of the medical profession is to ease pain, if acting to ease suffering a physician must introduce and follow a modality of treatment that may in fact hasten death, his actions are legally permissible so long as the understanding is maintained that the course of treatment is *only* for the relief of pain or associated distress.[123] This is a pre-eminently reasonable *modus operandi* for dealing with the double effect construct. Whether actions of this nature or constructions of the principle of double effect painlessly expedite death and thereby unwisely validate the traditional perception of passive euthanasia or (perhaps) passive suicide—more correctly termed "self-determination" in this chapter—and should accordingly be restricted or even forbidden socially and legally—will be examined in the following section.

LEGAL DISTINCTIONS

The legal distinction between acts and omission is made thusly:

> In the determination of the existence of a duty, there runs through much of the law a distinction between action and inaction.... There arose very early a difference, still deeply rooted in the law of negligence, between "misfeasance" and "nonfeasance"—that is to say, between active misconduct working positive injury to others and passive inaction or a failure to take steps to protect them from harm. The reason for the distinction may be said to lie in the fact that by 'misfeasance' the defendant has created a new risk of harm to the plaintiff, while by 'nonfeasance' he has at least made his situation no worse, and has merely failed to benefit him by interfering in his affairs...."
> Liability for "misfeasance" ... may extend to any person to whom

harm may reasonably be anticipated as a result of the defendant's conduct, or perhaps even beyond; while for 'nonfeasance' it is necessary to find some definite relation between the parties, of such a character that social duty justifies the imposition of a duty to act.[124]

It is argued, accordingly, that the distinction between assisting with the death of a patient and allowing him to die has a distinct parallel within the American legal system itself by the ways in which culpability is assigned for either "causing" or "permitting" harm to be inflicted upon others.[125] For, in those instances where an act can be found that caused a wrong or harm, once the agent who has brought about the harm is identified, liability is assessed.[126] Interestingly, with cases of omission, however, liability will not be imposed unless a "relationship" between the parties is established.[127]

The act of turning off an artificial respirator in use by a patient may be classified traditionally as either an act of commission or an act of omission.[128] Though a distinction may not be drawn easily here—because either action stems from the activity—the physician, if found to have committed an affirmative act of commission may be held liable for murdering the patient.[129] Crucial to the determination of the nature of the action would be a characterization of whether the act, itself, caused life to be terminated or was more properly considered as an omission to render aid to sustain life—thus permitting it to end. The operative verbs here are "caused" and "permitting."[130] In "acting" or "causing," an act of intercession is made to terminate life; while with acts of "omitting" or "permitting," a simple failure to intercede in a course of action to preserve life is recognized with the end-result that death is permitted to occur.[131] In determining legally whether the act of turning off a hypothetical respirator is one of commission or omission, consideration must also be given to the very doctor-patient relationship (as opposed to a non-associated one), patient reliance and reasonable expectation as well as the actual physical act of turning off the respirator, itself, and the circumstances surrounding it.[132]

It could be argued that the most crucial of all elements—motive—is the testing rod in aiding a determination of whether acts were those of commission or omission.[133] Accordingly, a deliberate act of killing—but one not done with a particularized motive or evil will—that is designed to allow the ending of life for a terminally ill patient and thus thereby relieve a life of suffering should not be classified as murder.[134] Inasmuch as no personal gain or good inures to the actor—but rather to the recipient of the immediate action—this would be another reason not to recognize the act as murder.[135] Noble intentions, however, are not always exculpatory. For example, if one subscribed to the belief of metempsychosis and decided to hasten another along toward the road to ultimate perfection before he became either tempted or corrupted with moral guilt, this act would surely be held to murder.[136]

Under one line of philosophical reasoning, acquiescing to a request for murder made by one fully conscious, who for physical or psychological reasons finds life unbearable and finds no other act suitable to bring a resolution to the quandry, would not be an act of murder; homicide, rather obviously. But, for a murder to be committed, there must be an infringement of rights. Here is seen but a simple and volitional release of the right to life.[137]

> ... if something is a right at all, then it can be given up; just as a gift, if it is a gift, can be renounced. Therefore, in cases where the quality of life has reached a certain subjective minimum, the individual has a right to give up that life, to request euthanasia. Consequently, in such cases euthanasia would be morally acceptable.[138]

Criminal Liability

For criminal liability to be imposed for not executing a duty owed, the leading American case hold that this duty must be,

> ... a legal duty, and not a mere moral obligation. It must be a duty imposed by law or by contract, and the omission to perform the duty must be the immediate and direct cause of death.[139]

Since the relationship between physicians and patient is basically contractual—arising from the nature of an offer and acceptance—a physician has no obligation to treat all comers. Only when treatment is undertaken does the law impose a duty on him to continue the level of treatment, in the absence of a contrary understanding, so long as the individual case required.[140] For the terminal patient desiring a swift, painless death, discharging the attending physician—in theory—terminates not only the physician's duty but also eliminates the primary basis for his criminal liability.[141] Therefore, the question of an imposition of criminal liability arises only in those cases where the physician has not been discharged or has failed to withdraw from a case with proper notice and thus, presumptively, the physician-patient relationship continues.[142] The physician may not seek a termination of this relationship by abandonment of the patient—for it is within this context that the possibility of criminal liability arises most generally.[143]

The history of the American case law of euthanasia presents an interesting record of a system that has prosecuted for the offense limitedly.[144] In fact, as early as 1916, the predominate view was that even when life is taken, with consent, in order to relieve either suffering or an "other greater calamity," and the resulting death is thus of meritorious character, such action would normally form the basis of a criminal prosection.[145] Yet, both judges and juries are reluctant to act affirmatively here.[146]

A survey of American case law reveals some twelve cases involving active euthanasia where only one resulted in an actional conviction for murder—with three others maintained for convictions for offenses less than murder, seven received acquittals and one failed because of no indictment.[147] In construing this same survey, one authority has noted that there were actually nine acquittals in all—with seven being allowed on the grounds of temporary insanity.[148] Observing that the standards for finding insanity are "tightening," he concluded that future acquittals of cases similar to these twelve may be more difficult to obtain.[149]

In the only case from the list of twelve that resulted in a conviction for murder, the plaintiff, Attorney John Noxon, was convicted of first degree murder and sentenced to death for the electrocution of his six-month old mongoloid son.[150] His sentence was subsequently commuted to life in prison, which was in turn reduced to six years.[151] The two cases involving physicians from the list revealed that the charges maintained against them were as a consequence of their efforts to ease the burden of interminable suffering for their patients by injecting them with potassium chloride[152] and air.[153] Neither of the physicians defended on the grounds that they were insane when they pursued this action.[154]

The International Perspective

An international incident that occurred in 1975 in Zurich, Switzerland, highlights the typical legal problem encountered with a policy of withdrawal of tubal feeding.[155] For, it was in January of that year a prominent Swedish physician, Peter Haemmerli, was accused of murder by starvation for failing to force feed unnamed terminally ill patients in a local hospital over a four-to-five-year period.[156] The charge—although no formal prosecution resulted since there had to be an allegation of a particular murder—was made as a consequence of a casual conversation by Dr. Haemmerli to a local politically aspiring city council member and designated health officer about the manner in which terminal patients were treated at the hospital where the doctor was on staff. More specifically, it was revealed that for an individual for example who had had a stroke, lapsed into a coma and after months had failed to gain consciousness and—in the opinion of the medical staff would never become conscious— the treatment followed was to discontinue tubal feeding, and proceed to administer a solution of salt and water which would prevent dehydration and maintain the normal chemical balance in the blood. Normally, the patient would die within several weeks as a result of starvation and without pain (in so far as anyone can determine, that is, a comatose person is immune from any associated type of pain during this course of treatment).[157]

Although accepted medical practice, the question must be raised as to the value and the humanness of letting people die without a semblance of dignity and in the manner as Dr. Haemmerli did. Does society *profit* from this type of action? What moral or ethical principles are validated as a consequence of undertakings of this nature—beneficence, respect for persons? No, sadly, the only position that is maintained is that of the *status quo*—a position or value that stresses the continuation of a practice or policy merely because it has been done so over the years. Contemporary times demand contemporary, thoughtful and humane responses to the critical issue of terminally ill patients, not lock-step repetitions of past follies.

In Holland, both the attitude about voluntary active euthanasia and its practice appear to be far different than anywhere else in the world.[158] In fact, the government has announced that it will structure legal guidelines under which euthanasia will be permitted.[159] It is unclear whether the guidelines will take the form of actual legislation or be set as administrative regulations.[160] Regardless of the final governmental approach, the present Dutch law prohibiting active euthanasia would remain and what would be done with this new approach would be to fashion various permissible exceptions to the law.[161]

The most famous open practitioner of voluntary active euthanasia appears to be Dr. Pieter Admiraal who is a physician at the Reiner de Graff General Hospital in Delft.[162] Once it is determined that one of the doctor's patients is dying—with a second opinion being obtained as to this fact—a team of other doctors, nurses and a priest or representative of the appropriate faith is assembled.[163] "Once a patient has repeatedly and lucidly requested euthanasia and the team have discussed the various alternatives of relief of pain or depression, the decision may be taken to go ahead."[164] Although case law does not require that any other parties than the physician and his patient be involved, as a safeguard the spouse or family is involved or at least advised of the decision.[165] Once the final decision is made, Dr. Admiraal follows one of two methods to implement it: a barbituate drip will be used that normally induces a state of unconsciousness within a few hours and death within six or eight hours or, in a few cases, some days later or a direct injection of barbituates and curare which also results in unconsciousness for the patient—but within a few minutes and death a few moments later.[166]

With an approximate population of fourteen million people, it is estimated in Holland that somewhere between six to ten thousand people a year (or some eight percent of the total number of deaths in the nation) are thought to die as a consequence of active voluntary euthanasia with the assistance of their physicians.[167] Currently, only about sixty actual cases are declared to be caused by euthanasia.[168] While each one has to be investigated by the local public prosecutor, should they then be prosecuted and should the physician in turn be found guilty, he would *not* be sentenced upon his conviction—thereby avoiding the establishment of a criminal record.[169]

A CONSTRUCTIVE PROPOSAL: RE-DEFINITION AND RE-EDUCATION

What is needed desperately in order to bring a contemporary sophistication—legal, medical, philosophical, ethical and moral—to the area of concern and investigation here is a strong definitional stance surrounding the term, "euthanasia" and "suicide"; quite simply, a re-education. More precisely, what is proposed is a change in the essential taxonomy of euthanasia as a word, concept, principle, attitude or legal action. Therefore, what has heretofore been recognized as acts of euthanasia of one form or other would be henceforth known as but acts of enlightened self-determination. Freed of the shackles of confusion and indecisiveness, actions undertaken within the context of an irreversible medical crisis or terminal illness[170] would be understood not as an act of autonomous rational suicide (or active euthanasia of oneself), or a refusal of treatment, but rather merely an act of enlightened self-determination. For the incapacitated or incompetent individual, the action taken on his behalf by a surrogate decision maker would be viewed similarly and the actions of these decision makers judged on their reasonableness and fairness to the terminal patient and his immediate family or extended family (assuming one exists).

This proposal would, in turn, begin to foster a new attitude toward death; one that would re-define the basic tasks of medicine as while not only recognizing old age as an honorable estate but that it is also unjust and inhumane to insist on an obligation being imposed upon old people suffering from a terminal illness or otherwise severely incapacitated to be forced to live through a period of miserable decline and painful helplessness.[171] The competent decision maker, at whatever age, suffering from a severe debilitating (terminal) disease, as well as the incompetent who is similarly situated and further inconvenienced by infancy, mental incompetence or unconsciousness, would also be accorded the privilege of holding first class citizenship; for the co-ordinate result of this new attitude about health care would be an unyielding recognition of the fact that a total right of personal autonomy is possessed by all.

Rational assisted suicide and all the varieties of euthanasia would no longer be considered. The major focus of all inquiry into actions previously classified as suicide or euthanasia would be simply: did the individual in question, exercising his powers of rational thinking, exercise an act of enlightened self-determination or autonomy. For the incompetent suffering from a similar terminal illness, the question to be answered would be: Did the surrogate decision maker, acting with rationality and humaneness, and thereby within the best interests of the terminal patient, or employing the principle of substituted judgment for that individual, exercise an act of enlightened self-determination. Obviously, the health care providers, and when brought into the matter, the courts, would themselves act under the presumption an individual within these circumstances or his duly appointed surrogate decision maker acted properly. It is realized that this position is a large quantum leap in not only thinking and hoped-for action, but it is an eminently fair and reasonable contemporary approach to an age-old problem. New wine in *new* wine bottles is the order of the day and of tomorrow as well.

ENDNOTES

1. M. KOHL, THE MORALITY OF KILLING 93 (1974).
2. See Chapter II, notes 98–155.

3. KASS, Man's Right to Die, 35 THE PHAROS 73, 74 (1972).

4. Id.

5. Id.

6. Ladd, Introduction, in ETHICAL ISSUES RELATING TO DEATH at 4 (J. LADD, ed. 1979).

7. Supra note 1 at 76.

8. Id. at 75, 76.

9. R. VEATCH, DEATH, DYING AND THE BIOLOGICAL REVOLUTION 77 (1976).

Positive euthanasia has been stated as doing something that ends life deliberately and is the form in which the issue of suicide is brought into question (as a voluntary or direct choice of death). The end-goal of both direct or positive and indirect or negative euthanasia is precisely the same—the end of a patient's life and a release from pointless misery and dehumanizing loss of bodily functions. Fletcher, In Defense of Suicide, in SUICIDE AND EUTHANASIA: THE RIGHTS OF PERSONHOOD 38 at 47 (S. Wallace, A. Eser eds. 1981).

10. Veatch, supra note 9.

11. Kuhse, The Case for Active Voluntary Euthanasia, 14 LAW, MED. & HEALTH CARE 145, 147 (1986).

12. Id.

13. Id.

14. Id.

15. Id.

16. Id.

17. R. VEATCH, DEATH, DYING AND THE BIOLOGICAL REVOLUTION 135 (1976).

See Richards, Constitutional Privacy, The Right to Die and The Meaning of Life: A Moral Analysis, 22 WILL. & MARY L. REV. 327 (1981).

18. M. KOHL, THE MORALITY OF KILLING 95 (1974).

19. Id. at 95–96.

20. Id. at 96.

21. Id. at 99.

22. Id.

23. Id. at 100.

24. K. KLUGE, THE PRACTICE OF DEATH 149 (1975).

25. M. KOHL, THE MORALITY OF KILLING 103, 106 (1974).

26. Id. at 107.

National attention was drawn to the poignancy and humaneness of euthanasia when—in its January 8, 1988, issue—the American Medical Association printed an anonymous column entitled, "It's Over Debbie," written by a physician who described the manner in which he deliberately injected a twenty year old young woman suffering from ovarian cancer with an overdose of morphine, 74 J.A.M.A. 272 (1988). Subsequently, citing confidentiality and First Amendment issues, the American Medical Association refused to provide the Cook County State Attorney's request to provide a grand jury in Chicago with the name of the physician who authored the column. Specter, AMA Won't Identify Mercy Killer, Wash. Post, Feb. 17, 1988, at A3, col. 1. The Chief Judge of the Cook County Court ruled later that no crime had been proved and dismissed a later grand jury subpoena demanding the physician author's identity. Wilkerson, Judge Stalls Inquiry into a Mercy Killing Case, N.Y. Times, Mar. 19, 1988, at 6, col. 1. See also, Wash. Post Health Mag., April 12, 1988, at 10, col. 1; Cohn, Saving Lives, Ending Lives, Wash. Post Health Mag., Mar. 1, 1988, at 13, col. 1.

27. E. KLUGE, THE PRACTICE OF DEATH 161 (1975).

28. Id.

29. Id.

30. Id.

31. Id. at 162.

32. Id.

33. Id. at 162.

34. Supra Ch. IV, notes 1–7.

35. McCormick, To Save or Let Die: The Dilemma of Modern Medicine in HOW BRAVE A NEW WORLD? at 339–349 (R. McCORMICK ed. 1981).

36. Rachels, Euthanasia, Killing and Letting Die in ETHICAL ISSUES RELATING TO DEATH at Ch. 7, p. 148 (J. LADD, ed. 1979).

See also, J. RACHELS, THE END OF LIFE (1986).

37. Appelbaum & Klein, Therefore Choose Death?, 81 COMMENTARY 23, 27 (1986).

38. Rachels, Euthanasia, Killing and Letting Die, supra.

For example, if someone were to see that an infant were drowning in a bathtub, would it make any difference whether an act of active or passive euthanasia were followed? It could be perceived "just as bad to let it drown as to push its head under water," for one action is as iniquitous as the other. Foot, Euthanasia in ETHICAL ISSUES RELATING TO DEATH 28, at 29 (J. LADD ed. 1979).

39. F. HARRON, J. BURNSIDE, & T. BEAUCHAMP, HEALTH AND HUMAN VALUES 48 (1983).

40. Id.

See also, Rachels, Active and Passive Euthanasia, 292 NEW ENG. J. MED. 78 (1975).

41. Id. at 42.

42. Id.

43. Id.

44. 140 MED. J. AUST. 431 (Oct. 1981).

45. Kuhse, Euthanasia—again, 142 MED. J. AUST. 610, 611 (1985).

46. Id.

47. Fearing condonation or actual use of "poisons or similar lethal agents" upon request by a patient would "risk serious abuse," the President's Commission for the Study of Ethical Problems in Medicine and Biomedical and Behavioral Research refused to sanction such usage. See DECIDING TO FOREGO LIFE–SUSTAINING TREATMENT: ETHICAL, MEDICAL AND LEGAL ISSUES IN TREATMENT

DECISIONS, 62 *passim* (1983). Yet, the Commission did recognize the treatment refusals for dying patients should be honored. Id. at 63.

The Law Reform Commission of Canada has concluded euthanasia should not be legalized because such a condonation would severely weaken respect for all human life. Rather, it suggests a better answer to the sufferings of terminally ill would be to develop more effective palliative care and to search for equally effective pain control therapies. Report 20, EUTHANASIA, AIDING SUICIDE AND CESSATION TREATMENT, REPORT OF THE LAW REFORM COMMISSION OF CANADA 17, 18, 21, 31 (1983). The Commission did recognize that patients are autonomous decision makers and, acting within this role, have a right to make a decision regarding the discontinuation of treatment either already in progress or not to even commence any type of treatment at all; and that this expression of one's will is but a simple question of fact. Id.

48. Kuhse, The Case for Active Voluntary Euthanasia, 14 LAW, MED. & HEALTH CARE 145, 147 (1986).

49. Id.

50. Amundsen, The Physician's Obligation to Prolong Life: A Medical Duty Without Classical Roots, 8 HASTINGS CENTER RPT. 23 (Aug. 1978).

51. Id. at 27.

52. Id.

53. Id. at 25.

54. Id.

55. Id. at 27, 28.

56. Supra note 614 at 27.

57. Id.

58. Id.

59. President's Commission for the Study of Ethical Problems in Medicine and Biomedical and Behavioral Research, DECIDING TO FOREGO LIFE-SUSTAINING TREATMENT: ETHICAL, MEDICAL, AND LEGAL ISSUES IN TREATMENT DECISIONS at 300–307 (1983).

See, Sometimes Extending Life Only Prolongs Death, N.Y. TIMES, Sept. 23, 1984, at 6E, col. 1.

60. Id. at 305.

61. Id.

62. Id. Emphasis provided.

63. Id. Emphasis provided.

See Hansen, Right to Die: A Consensus is Emerging with Assistance of Catholic Theologians, NAT'L CATHOLIC RPTR, Dec. 11, 1987, at 1 col. 1.

64. Id.

65. Id. Emphasis provided.

66. Id.

67. See generally, Smith, *Triage:* Endgame Realities, 1 J. CONTEMP. H. L. & POL'Y 143 (1985).

One prominent Jesuit theologian, Fr. Edwin J. Healey, has implied that the maximum amount of money that could be expended on an ordinary course of treatment *before* it became extraordinary, was $2,000.00. Kelly, The Duty of Using Artificial Means of Preserving Life, 11 Theological Studies 203 at 206 f.n. 9 citing Fr. Healey (1950).

68. Supra note 59 at 307.

69. R. McCormick, NOTES ON MORAL THEOLOGY, 1965 through 1980, at 565 (1981).

70. J. CHILDRESS, WHO SHOULD DECIDE: PATERNALISM IN HEALTH CARE 166 (1982).

71. Hilfiker, Allowing the Debilitated to Die: Facing Our Ethical Choices, 308 N. ENG. J. MED. 716 (Mar. 24, 1983).

72. Childress, When Is It Morally Justifiable to Discontinue Medical Nutrition and Hydration? in BY NO EXTRAORDINARY MEANS at 81 (J. LYNN, ed. 1986).

73. Id.

74. Smith, Quality of Life, Sanctity of Creation: Palliative or Apotheosis?, 63 NEB. L. REV. 707, 734 (1984).

75. G. SMITH, GENETICS, ETHICS AND THE LAW 1–4 (1981).

76. Supra note 74.

77. Supra note 75.

78. Supra note 74 at 738.

79. The ultimate morality of an action or inaction in cases of this nature being considered here can never be evaluated properly without reference to the quality of life being extended by the heroic measures. G. WILL, When Homicide is Noble, in THE MORNING AFTER: AMERICAN SUCCESSES AND EXCESSES 1981–86 at 84, 85 (1986).

80. Supra note 75 at 9.

81. Beall, Mercy for the Terminally Ill Cancer Patient, 249 J.A.M.A. 2883 (June 3, 1983).

82. 1982 A.M.A. JUDICIAL COUNCIL CURRENT OPINIONS, Am. Med. Assoc. 9–10 (1982); President's Commission for the Study of Ethical Problems in Medicine and Biomedical and Behavioral Research, DECIDING TO FOREGO LIFE-SUSTAINING TREATMENT: ETHICAL, MEDICAL, AND LEGAL ISSUES IN TREATMENT DECISIONS at 288 (1983).

83. Kelly, the Duty of Using Artificial Means of Preserving Life, 11 THEO-LOGICAL STUDIES 203, 206 (1950).

84. Id. at 207.

85. H. ENGELHARDT, JR., THE FOUNDATIONS OF BIOETHICS 307 (1986).

86. G. KELLY, MEDICO–MORAL PROBLEMS 129 (1958).

87. D. MAGUIRE, DEATH BY CHOICE 123 (1975).

Only when there is hope of health (*si sit spes salutis*) or where hope of recovery appeared (*ubi spes affulget convalescendi*) is treatment required. Futile treatments (*nemo ad inutile*) or treatments that only postponed death or blunted briefly the illness (*parum pro nihilo reputatur moralitier*) are not required to be undertaken. An obligation to accept treatment is defeated if the at-risk individual has an aversion to the particular form of treatment (*horror magnus*). H. ENGELHARDT, JR., THE FOUNDATIONS OF BIOETHICS 332, f.n. 122 (1986).

88. H. ENGELHARDT, JR., THE FOUNDATIONS OF BIOETHICS 235 (1986).
89. Id.
90. Supra note 83 at 214.
91. Id. at 210 quoting J. V. Sullivan, Catholic Teaching on the Morality of Euthanasia.
    Another fascinating case is to be found in considering the duty to use or administer insulin with reference to a patient who has both diabetes and cancer. The patient would be required to use the insulin because it is the normal, ordinary manner to combat or stabilize the diabetes. The interesting problem here is whether one who suffers from two lethal diseases is obligated to pursue ordinary treatments in order to check one when there is no hope of checking the other disease that is lethal. Stated otherwise, given the presence of the terminable cancer, can insulin injections be regarded as a reasonable hope of success? Should the diseases be considered separately or would it be better to evaluate the total patient condition? It is argued that for the clear duty to use insulin to exist, two factors must exist: it must be both an ordinary means as well as offer a reasonable hope of success. Obviously, the presence of cancer casts some serious doubt on this second factor. Id. at 216.
92. 380 N.E. 2d 134, 137 n. 7 (Mass. App. Ct. 1978).
93. 373 Mass. 728, 370 N.E. 2d 417, 424 (1977). Emphasis supplied.
94. 70 N.J. 10, 335 A. 2d 647, 668, *cert. denied* 429 U.S. 922 (1976). Emphasis supplied.
95. Ramsey, Euthanasia and Dying Well Enough, 44 LINACRE Q. 43 (1977).
96. Id.
    See also, Ramsey, Prolonged Dying: Not Medically Indicated, 6 HASTINGS CENTER RPT. 16 (Feb. 16, 1976).
97. R. VEATCH, DEATH, DYING AND THE BIOLOGICAL REVOLUTION 110 (1976).
98. Id.
99. Id.
100. Id. at 112.
    See generally, R. McCORMICK, HOW BRAVE A NEW WORLD, Ch. 21 (1981).
101. CHILDRESS, WHO SHOULD DECIDE: PATERNALISM IN HEALTH CARE 166 (1982).
102. Id.
103. Id.
104. Id.
105. R. VEATCH, A THEORY OF MEDICAL ETHICS 37, 39 (1981).
106. Id. at 39.
107. Martin, Suicide and Self Sacrifice in SUICIDE: THE PHILOSOPHICAL ISSUES 48 at 58 (M. BATTIN, D. MAYO eds. 1980).
108. Supra note 160.
    Stated more specifically, the action from which evil results is good or indifferent in itself (e.g., administering a pain killer); only the good consequences of the action must be intended (e.g., relief of the patient's suffering)—the evil effect (e.g., the possible death of the patient due to the administration of a sufficiently large

dose will *surely* kill the pain but *might* cause death) is sincerely not intended; the good effect must not be produced by means of the evil effect (the relief of the patient's suffering must not be produced by the patient's death; therefore, the dosage of pain-killers must sincerely be thought of as sufficient to ease the pain without also surely causing the patient's death—the question then becomes how certain can one be about the possible occurrence of the evil effect before the principle is violated; otherwise it would be a means to the good effect before the principle is violated; otherwise it would be a means to the good effect and would be intended; and there must be proportionately grave reason for allowing the evil to occur. R. McCORMICK, HOW BRAVE A NEW WORLD? 412–429 (1981).

See also, President's Commission for the Study of Ethical Problems in Medicine and Biomedical and Behavioral Research, DECIDING TO FOREGO LIFE–SUSTAINING TREATMENT: ETHICAL, MEDICAL, AND LEGAL ISSUES IN TREATMENT DECISIONS at 80, n. 10 (1983).

109. Supra note 106 at 39.

110. Id. at 235.

Where treatment offered to extend life would be unreasonably burdensome or simply useless to a terminally ill patient, the Principle would permit non treatment. Id. at 40.

111. Louisell, Euthanasia and Biathanasia, 22 CATH. UNIV. L. REV. 723, 742 (1973).

112. Id.

113. Id.

114. Smith, *Triage:* Endgame Realities, 1 J. CONTEMP. H. L. & POL'Y 143 (1985).

115. Engelhardt, Suicide and The Cancer Patient, 36 CA–A Cancer Journal for Clinicians 105, 108 (1986).

116. Id.

117. Id.

118. Id.

119. Id.

120. C. SAUNDERS, M. BAINES, LIVING WITH DYING: THE MANAGEMENT OF TERMINAL DISEASE 4 (1983).

121. Id.

122. Id.

123. Id.

The double effect principle was validated in the case of *Rex v. Bodkin-Adams* (1957). Here, Dr. Joh Bodkin-Adams was acquitted of murder after having administered narcotics that apparently caused the death of his patient. The judge held (in this unreported case) that a physician who administers narcotics in order to relieve pain is not guilty of murder merely because the measures he takes incidentally shorten life. O. RUSSELL, FREEDOM TO DIE 255 (1977).

124. W. PROSSER, THE LAW OF TORTS §56 at 373–74 (15th ed. 1984).

125. Fletcher, Prolonging Life, 42 WASH. L. REV. 909 (1967).

126. Id. at 1009, 1012.

127. Id.

128. See R. WILLIAMS, TO LIVE AND TO DIE: WHEN, WHY AND HOW (1973); Fletcher, Legal Aspects of the Decision Not to Prolong Life, 203 J.A.M.A. 65 (1968).

129. Comment, The Right to Die, 7 HOUSTON L. REV. 654, 659 (1970).

130. Fletcher, supra note 128.

131. Id.

132. Supra note 125.

Truly, the bounds of moral judgment are strained to the point of collapse when an ultimate decision is sought as to whether switching off a respirator is an act of active euthanasia or merely passive euthanasia! Rachels, Active and Passive Euthanasia, 292 NEW ENG. J. MED. 78 (1975).

In a 1983 California case, *Barber v. Superior Court of Los Angeles County,* 147 Cal. App. 3d 1006, 195 Cal. Rptr. 484, the court recognized that there was a difference between killing and letting die and that actions by two doctors in turning off a respirator of a patient who was vegetative, with permission from the patient's wife, was not an act of killing.

133. E. KLUGE, THE PRACTICE OF DEATH 171 (1975).

134. Id.

135. Id.

136. Id.

137. Id.

138. Id.

139. *People v. Beardsley,* 150 Mic. 206, 113 N.W. 1128, 1129 (1907).

140. Survey, Euthanasia: Criminal, Tort, Constitutional and Legislative Considerations, 48 NOTRE DAME L. REV. 1202, 1207 (1973).

141. Id. at 1208.

142. Id.

143. Id.

A new and novel tort action for *wrongful living* has been proposed recently. Under the proposal, the tort would be recognized as personal and hence redressed only by the individual whose right to die was compromised; or, if that individual should die subsequently, by his representative on a survival basis. If the interferring treatment is made and thereupon the patient lives, the interference with the right to die involves compensation for the living. Contrariwise, if the interferring treatment causes death earlier than non treatment, then there is a clear, causal connection between the interference and the loss: permanent death. Accordingly, wrongful death damages to the beneficiaries of the decedent would be appropriate; but damages could be calculated for that period of time by which the life was shortened by the treatment. Oddi, The Tort of Interference with the Right to Die: The Wrongful Living Cause of Action, 75 GEO. L. J. 625, 641 (1980).

See also, Furrow, Damage Remedies and Institutional Reform: The Right to Refuse Treatment, 12 LAW, MED. & HEALTH CARE 152 (1982).

144. Survey, Euthanasia: Criminal, Tort, Constitutional and Legislative Considerations, 48 NOTRE DAME L. REV. 1202, 1213 (1973).

145. Id.

146. Id.

147. Id. at 1213, f.n. 82.

148. R. VEATCH, DEATH, DYING AND THE BIOLOGICAL REVOLUTION 79 (1976).

149. Id. See generally, MacKinnon, Euthanasia and Homicide, 26 CRIM. L. Q. 483 (1984).

150. *Commonwealth v. Noxon,* 319 Mass. 495, 66 N.E. 2d 814 (1946).

151. Supra note 144, at 1214, f.n. 86.

152. R. VEATCH, DEATH, DYING AND THE BIOLOGICAL REVOLUTION 78 (1976).

See the June, 1973, account of the case of a fifty-nine year old Long Island man dying of cancer whose attending physician, Dr. Vincent A. Montemorano, was indicted for taking the patient's life by injecting potassium chloride into him — but was found innocent of the action at trial. Id.

153. R. VEATCH, supra at 79, 80.

In New Hampshire in 1950, Dr. Herman Sander was charged with committing the murder of Mrs. Abbie Brown, who was dying of cancer, by giving her intravenous injections of air — and he was acquitted at trial. Id.

154. Id. at 80.

A brief analysis and listing of the nine or so widely publicized mercy-killing court cases (not officially reported) against physicians is found in O. RUSSELL, FREEDOM TO DIE, 255–256, 260, 329 (Rev. ed. 1977).

In a particularly famous English case in 1957, involving the charge of murder against Dr. John Bodkin-Adams for allegedly administering narcotics to relieve pain, the court found Dr. Adams not guilty of murder even though the course of treatment that was administered incidentally shortened the life of the decedent. Id. at 255, 329. See, supra, note 123.

In 1983, two physicians were found innocent of committing murder when they disconnected a respirator and stopped artificial feeding and hydration for a patient — these actions all being done with written approval from the patient's spouse. *Barber v. Superior Court of Los Angeles County,* 147 Cal. App. 3d 1006, 195 Cal. Rptr. 484 (1983).

155. Culliton, The Haemmerli Affair: Is Passive Euthanasia Murder?, 90 SCIENCE 1271 (1975).

See also, O. RUSSELL, FREEDOM TO DIE 350, 351 (1977 rev. ed.).

156. Id.

157. Calliton at 1272.

158. Cody, Dutch Weigh Legalizing Euthanasia: Gap Cited Between Law and Practice, WASH. POST, Mar. 16, 1987, at 1, col. 3.

159. Id.

See Schepens, Euthanasia: Our Own Future, 3 Issues LAW & MED. 371, 377 (1988) for the listing of the guidelines.

160. Id.

161. Id.

The British Medical Association currently has an eight member working committee studying euthanasia. Although at present the BMA condemns active involuntary or active voluntary euthanasia, in cases of passive euthanasia there are mixed feelings. Appelyard, The Last Appointment, The Sunday Times Mag. (London), June 17, 1987, at 13, 22.

Switzerland, Uruguay, Peru, Japan and Germany allow a physician the right to comply with a patient's request for death medication under certain circumstances. It is not a punishable crime for a physician to assist with a suicide if his motivation is altruistic. M. HEIFETZ, THE RIGHT TO DIE 96 (1975).

162. Appelyard, supra.

163. Id. at 13, 16.

As early as 1958, it was advocated by an eminent Cambridge University professor that the least cumbersome approach to the euthanasia problem was to employ referees or committees to determine the validity of requests for voluntary active euthanasia and to similarly relieve an assisting physician of all liability if he acted in good faith. G. WILLIAMS, THE SANCTITY OF LIFE AND THE CRIMINAL LAW, Ch. 8 at 340 (1958).

164. Appelyard, supra note 161 at 13.

165. Id. at 16.

166. Id.

167. Id. at 13.

168. Id. at 18.

169. Id.

In 1984, Maria Barendregt—a 94-year-old—was rendered helpless by her old age. Her mind was intact although she had extended bouts of unconsciousness; and she was unable to care for herself. Her physician acquiesced to her demand for euthanasia and adjudicated, the case held that proximity to death is not a necessary condition for allowing euthanasia. Id. at 20.

In the celebrated *De Terp* case, a physician and nurse working in an old person's home euthanized three of their patients there and were found guilty of murder and sentenced to a year of imprisonment—only upon appeal, to be freed. Id. 20.

170. This term would be defined as "an illness in which, on the basis of the best available diagnostic criteria and in the light of available therapies, a reasonable estimation can be made prospectively and with a high probability that a person will die within a relatively short time." Bayer, Callahan, Fletcher, et al, The Care of The Terminally Ill: Morality and Economics, 309 NEW ENG. J. MED. 1490, 1491 (1983).

171. See, Barrington, Apologia for Suicide in SUICIDE: THE PHILOSOPHICAL ISSUES at 90, 99, 100 (M. BATTIN, D. MAYO eds. 1980).

Chapter V

ORDERS NOT TO RESUSCITATE AND THE WITHDRAWAL OR WITHHOLDING OF TREATMENT

INCREMENTAL STEPS TOWARD PASSIVE EUTHANASIA

In 1973, the National Conference on Standards for Cardiopulmonary Resuscitation and Emergency Cardiac Care sought to establish a procedure which would allow physicians to indicate further medical treatment was not advantageous to particular patients in their care. Accordingly, the Conference suggested that a rather simple "order not to resuscitate" (ONTR) could be indicated in the progress notes or chart for the distressed patient and, in turn, communicated to the hospital staff.[1] To be distinguished from other forms of medical care that terminate pre-existing patient support systems such as the discontinuance of respirators, ONTR includes instructions not only not to use inotropic or vasopressor drugs that increase cardiac contractility and maintain blood pressure, but to not initiate cardiopulmonory resuscitation (CPR).[2] Orders not to resuscitate are ofter referred to as "no codes"—for they normally stipulate no emergency is to be given when cardiac or respiratory failure occurs.[3]

The inherent problems associated with the 1973 Cardiopulmonary Resuscitation and Emergency Care Conference Report on ONTR's are today—as real and complex as they were then. The central issues are tied to not only carefully determining with reasonable accuracy when an illness is terminal and when continued medical treatment contravenes the best interest of a terminally ill patient but whether principles of *triage*, or the efficient and maximum allocation of scarce medical resources—together with quality of life factors—should be evaluated in the deliberative process.[4]

The result of what has been termed, "the growing medicalization of death," is quite simply that human acts of intervention have nearly totally replaced natural processes.[5] Indeed, what with almost daily dis-

119

coveries of "miracle drugs," the perfection of new surgical routines and the development of new sophisticated mechanical mechanisms designed to assist or relieve normal bodily processes, illness—as such—can no longer be thought of as having a natural course of progressive development.[6] Thus, sadly, while heretofore pneumonia had to be regarded as the dear friend of the elderly ill patients and cardiopulmonary seizure was an almost certain guarantee of death, now frenzied actions of a "Code Blue Trauma Team" can be witnesses almost daily in any metropolitan hospital as the team races to, as the case merits, jump-start hearts with electric paddles and drugs and reinflate lungs with artificial pumps.[7] Today, death is no longer a family residential occurrence; rather it has been moved to a hospital or some type of health-care institution.[8]

The patient's autonomy or right of self-determination in health care issues must always be balanced against the same professional autonomy of a physician. Thus, no force or coercion can be exerted to compel a physician to proceed with treatment for a patient who has rejected resuscitation if that physician considers a provision for patient resuscitation to be an ethical, moral or professional obligation.[9] An important recognition of this professional autonomy for the physician must be allowed through maintenance of an option for him to transfer care of the terminal or at-risk patient.[10]

When courts are presented with a typical DNR case, they normally will utilize a balancing test that balances the patient's qualified right to refuse treatment against two other factors: the prognosis for the patient and the degree to which the DNR order will be invasive to bodily integrity, with state interest weakening and the individual privacy right strengthening as the prognosis for recovery lessens and the degree of bodily invasion increases.[11] Accordingly, in those cases where invasive treatment such as surgery or dialysis is dictated, the pervasive judicial attitude has been to uphold the patient's right to refuse treatment—even though there may well be a favorable patient prognosis.[12] The few number of courts that have considered ONTR's have realized the high invasive nature of cardiopulmonary resuscitation and approved them.[13]

THE 1976 MASSACHUSETTS GENERAL HOSPITAL PROTOCOL

In 1976, the Massachusetts General Hospital announced formally—although it had been in effect for some six months—its protocol on

"Optimum Care for Hopelessly Ill Patients" where the first step in the process of determining the level of care given to the critically ill (namely, the classification of their probability of survivability or, salvageability) was set forth.[14] Consistent with the time-honored principle of *triage*,[15] four classifications are listed: Class A, where "maximal therapeutic effort without reservation" will be given; Class B, where the same level of effort is given, but "with daily evaluation because probability of survival is questionable; Class C, where "selective limitation of therapeutic measures" is followed (here orders not to resuscitate or to withhold antibiotics that would otherwise arrest or cure pneumonia might normally be given); and Class D, "where all therapy can be discontinued," and would be normally only for patients suffering brain death or have no chance of regaining "cognitive and sapient."[16]

A permanent hospital committee on the optimum treatment of the hopelessly ill is in place when professional medical difference of opinion arises regarding treatment of a terminal patient. Thus, while the primary or "responsible physician" has full authority over the treatment of his patient (which includes the right not to seek the committee's advice at all or to reject it once given), the final authority would appear mitigated by further provisions within the guidelines allowing the director of intensive care to go directly to the chief of service and empanel the committee—regardless of whether the primary physician wishes to pursue this course.[17] It is thought that a physician would have to be particularly foolhardy or, in the alternative, courageous to act against the institutional judgment of his peers—regardless of the decision to treat, withdraw or withhold.

Institutional efforts of this nature present a model for effective and principled decision making. They also structure a verifiable process for evaluating the costs and benefits of treatment and non-treatment and thereby aid not only the health care providers in their decision making, but also the family members or surrogate decision makers who are advised, consulted or approve the ultimate decision.

The New York State Task Force on Life and the Law Statutory Proposal

In April, 1986, the New York State Task Force on Life and the Law issued its study of Orders Not to Resuscitate,[18] and proposed a model legislative scheme—from which in fact grew subsequent legislation—that will not only provide clear and comprehensive guidelines for decision making, but establish a strong mechanism for arbitration of challenges to decisions of this nature.[19] A number of major policies are embodied in this legislation which are germane to the present issue under consideration and which go far toward clarifying the medico-legal use of an order not to resuscitate. Thus, an analysis of the legislation, itself, is necessary.

While affirming the present presumption under existing law that all patients admitted to a hospital consent to cardiopulmonary resuscitation (CPR) in the event of an incident of cardiac or respiratory arrest, the legislation makes provision for consent for the withholding of CPR or the issuance of an order not to resuscitate in all hospitals and residential health care facilities in the State of New York.[20] Subject to a narrow therapeutic exception, an attending physician must obtain the consent of a patient with decisional authority prior to issuing a DNR order.[21] This decision by the patient in a hospital may be either expressed orally or—prior to or during hospitalization—in writing.[22]

Before the issuance of a DNR order, the attending physician must first obtain the contemporaneous consent of a patient with decisional capacity.[23] If, at the time of the issuance of such an order the at-risk patient lacks capacity—but had previously stated his wish in writing—to forego CPR, the writing will constitute consent to the issuance of the order.[24] Interestingly, and wisely, the legislation recognizes a narrow therapeutic exception which permits a physician to obtain consent to a DNR order from another person on behalf of the patient. This exception is premised on the fact that isolated circumstances may occur where a patient's capacity might be jeopardized and immediate injury occur from an actual discussion about resuscitation.[25] Although injury is not defined, the Task Force cited two examples of situations where discussion would be inadvisable: where a patient has an arrythmia for whom such a discussion could trigger cardiac arrest and where a patient is in a severe state of paranoic depression or has suicidal tendencies.[26]

Unless it is determined that an adult patient lacks capacity—not competence—to make a decision about resuscitation, the presumption is maintained that every adult is entitled to make a decision about resuscitation.[27] The "competence standard" relates usually to an individual's ability to make all decisions, while the "capacity standard" is tied to an assessment of one's ability to make a specific decision about resuscitation.[28] In those cases where a patient is without capacity to make a decision of this type or order, the attending physician is required to obtain the necessary consent from a surrogate, or substitute decision maker where such an individual is both available as well as willing and competent to speak for the patient.[29] Provision is made for patients with capacity to designate an individual to act for and on their behalf if they are expected to lack capacity at the time the decision must be made.[30]

One of four medical conditions must be in existence and a written determination made thereof by a physician before a surrogate decision maker may consent to the issuance of a DNR order for a patient lacking capacity.[31] The four conditions are finding that: 1) the patient is terminally ill; 2) irreversibly comatose or permanently unconscious; 3) medically futile and 4) resuscitation would impose an extraordinary burden on the patient in light of the patient's medical condition or the expected outcome of resuscitation.[32] The basis of the surrogate's decision here is tied to a determination of the patient's known wishes or religious and moral beliefs. If these wishes or beliefs are either unknown or not ascertainable, then the basis will be the patient's best interests.[33]

In those cases where a patient is lacking in capacity to make a DNR decision and a proper surrogate is unavailable, in order not to resuscitate can still be given if one of two conditions are met: a determination is made by two physicians that it would be medically futile to undertake the act or, based on clear and convincing evidence of either the patient's known wishes or in the absence thereof, a finding of the patient's best interests directs the issuance of a court order for a DNR.[34]

Before issuing a DNR order for a minor, under the legislation, the attending physician must first obtain the consent of such a minor's parent or legal guardian.[35] But if the attending physician, in consultation with the parents of the at-risk minor, determines the minor does have decisional capacity, then the minor's consent to the issuance of a DNR order must be obtained.[36]

The consent to the issuance of a DNR order is narrow and confined only to cardiopulmonary resuscitation; it *does not* authorize an extension of consent to withhold or withdraw medical treatment.[37] The legislation also sets out a procedure for revoking a DNR order and directs, simply, that the patient make a written or oral declaration "or by any other act evidencing a specific intent to revoke such consent or assent" to a physician or to a nurse at the treating hospital.[38] For the surrogate, parent or legal guardian, a similar procedure for revocation is provided.[39] Once the revocation of consent is obtained, it is to be entered immediately in the patient's chart and notification given to the hospital staff of the revocation and cancellation.[40]

Section Thirteen of this legislation mandates all hospitals and residential health care facilities to establish a dispute mediation system whereby all disagreements arising among the decision makers (i.e., patients, physicians, family members, etc.) participating in the resuscitation decision may be aired. The mediation system allows *any* party to the controversy to come before it and, at the same time, reserves to all parties the right to seek judicial relief in the event the matter is not resolved. Once a dispute is brought before the mediation service, the issuance of a DNR is stayed automatically for either seventy-two hours or until the conclusion of the mediation process—whichever occurs first.[41]

Judicial review of actions allowed under the legislation may be sought essentially by either the patient, attending physician, hospital, the facility director if the patient was transferred, any personal surrogate, the parents, non-custodial parent or legal guardian of a minor patient.[42] Even though provision is made for a required grace period of seventy-two hours once mediation has begun over a dispute regarding a DNR, the actual patient is not required to observe this period—but "may commence action for relief with respect to any dispute under this article at any time."[43]

For the physicians and other health care providers who comply in good faith with a DNR order or—contrariwise—resuscitate a patient for whom an order has been issued because of their unawareness of the order or because, again, in good faith, believed the order has been revoked, provision is made for a grant of civil and criminal immunity.[44] Equal protection from liability is also extended to persons designated to act for the patient who consents or declines to consent in good faith to the issuance of a DNR order.[45] Finally, it is stipulated in the legislation that no life insurance policy will be impaired or invalidated as a consequence of a DNR order nor can any person require or prohibit the issuance of a DNR order as either a condition for being insured or receiving health care services.[46]

To date, this proposal is the most balanced and comprehensive effort to both define, strengthen, and stabilize the rights, authority and protections afforded not only the at-risk patient, but his family, surrogate decision makers and health care providers who all participate—at one level or other—in the issuance of orders not to resuscitate. As such, it provides a vital structure for principled decision making, a blueprint for subsequent state response and a framework for achieving a national construct for response to this most critical area of contemporary medico-legal concern.

Unresolved Questions

A number of unresolved questions may be posited regarding the continued development and application of DNR's: 1.) Will new and more effective procedures be developed that will involve patients directly in do not resuscitate orders *before* they become moribund? 2.) Will prognosticative techniques be advanced to the point where identification of patients for whom resuscitation is done with a certainty instead of the current practice that allows only broad categorical designation? 3.) Since current studies show cancer — instead of cardiac disease and old age — is the most likely predictor of DNR status, does this represent a danger-point in subsequent efforts that might bias or pre-dispose the issuance of a DNR? 4.) What should be done with meeting the demands of families who insist all measure of life-sustaining treatment be done for the mori-bund patient, who — himself — has never expressed himself on the issue when such actions would be already futile? 5.) Should a level of concern be raised that as a consequence of anticipated greater specificity and detail for DNR policies at hospitals, broader categories of non-treatment decisions might become acceptable? 6.) How far should needs to contain the level of health costs through rationing of expensive and scarce interventions be considered in issuing DNR's?[47]

The complicated and often competing vectors of force or dynamics in non-treatment decisions must be understood and dealt with; and this is surely no simple task in a pluralistic society where a high level of consciousness exists regarding health care.[48] The courts can only go as far, and with as much clarity, as the medical profession is willing to provide it with an information base for its decision making. Of course, ideally, the judiciary should not ever intrude into the doctor-patient or familial sphere of decision making privacy. Perhaps this is too much to expect, given the vast amount of confusion regarding the "science" of orders not to resuscitate. The medical profession has everything to gain from efforts to control itself and define the parameters of its actions here. Its input into legislative proposals such as the New York Study are a laudable effort to bring clarity and structure to this area of concern and thereby hopefully prevent judicial intrusiveness.

THE AMERICAN MEDICAL ASSOCIATION'S GUIDELINES FOR WITHHOLDING OR WITHDRAWING LIFE-SUSTAINING TREATMENT

When Americans died in 1950, the majority died at home with their families and local physicians in attendance.[49] Now, as observed previously, death has become "medicalized" with the result that human interventions replace natural processes and thereby prolong life in one form or other.[50] With a growing array of high-powered life support techniques and so-called "miracle" drugs, death is but another matter of human choice and one laden with ethical complexities.[51] Presently, of the approximately five thousand, five hundred Americans who die each day, eight percent do so "wired and incubated, in an institution where the expensive technology is arrayed and controlled by specialists who likely know little about the patient beyond the medical problem."[52] Perhaps, in recognition of this phenomena, a 1985 Louis Harris poll of one thousand, two hundred and fifty-four adults disclosed the fact that eighty-five percent of them were of the opinion that a terminally ill patient "ought to be able to tell his doctor to let him die": and eighty-two percent supported the notion of withdrawing nasogastric (feeding) tubes if the at-risk patient directs such action.[53]

A poll sponsored by the American Medical Association—the results of which were released November 28, 1986—showed that nearly three of four Americans or seventy-three percent of the one thousand, five hundred and ten respondents in this survey, favor "withdrawing life support systems, including food and water, from hopelessly ill or irreversibly comatose patients if they or their family request it."[54] Fifteen percent of the respondents opposed this option and twelve percent expressed uncertainty.[55] Interestingly, seventy percent of those younger than sixty-five favored the proposal, as did sixty-four percent of those sixty-five or older. Twenty percent of the older group said they were unsure—compared with ten percent of the younger group. The withdrawal of life support systems was more likely to be favored by individual respondents having at least a high school education as well as by those whose annual income was more than $10,000.[56]

On March 15, 1986, the Council on Ethical and Judicial Affairs of the American Medical Association issued Guidelines for Withholding or Withdrawing Life Prolonging Medical Treatment for Terminally Ill or

Irreversibly Comatose Patients,[57] which in essence recognize that—ethically—a physician may withdraw "all means of life-prolonging medical treatment," including food and water, from patients who are terminally ill or who are in irreversible comas.[58] This policy statement is totally consistent with the conclusion of the President's Commission for the Study of Ethical Problems in Medicine and Biomedical and Behavioral Research that artificial feeding should be regarded as a treatment decision, and not mandated except where the benefits to be gained therefrom outweigh the burdens.[59]

Many individuals choose to make an emotional distinction between respirators and feeding tubes even though both are means of life support for comatose patients.[60] Somehow, an intravenous line is not only more familiar but less intrusive to a number of people than does an artificial respirator.[61] Interestingly, in what no doubt has become the most distinguished case involving a withholding of medical treatment, *In re Quinlan*,[62] Karen Ann Quinlan's family maintained a successful legal action to have her artificial respirator disconnected; but they declined to seek judicial approval of a withdrawal of nutritional support from her,[63] and Karen "lived" for ten years in a coma.

While it has been suggested that the withdrawal of nutritional support from a terminally ill or irreversibly comatose patient is dangerously close to murder,[64] and that soon guidelines might include the exclusion of "severely senile, the very old and decrepit, and maybe even young, profoundly retarded children,"[65] the AMA statement declares specifically that "the physicians should not intentionally cause death."[66] Since the Council position is no way binding, physicians who disagree with it are free to follow the dictates of their own conscience.[67]

Dr. Russel H. Patterson, Jr., Chairman of Neurosurgery at the New York University-Cornell Medical Center and a past president of the American Association of Neurological Surgeons, suggested that there is "a rather large jump between letting someone die and killing someone."[68] He continued by stating that withdrawing extraordinary life supports from those who have no hope of ever regaining consciousness is often the most humane treatment available.[69]

> After a while—maybe weeks or months of seeing the patient with no concept of the present, no memory of the past and no hope for the future—a lot of families say, "Why does this have to go on? What's the purpose?"[70]

The AMA policy acknowledges that while the physicians social commitment is to both sustain life and relieve suffering, these duties may conflict with each other from time to time. When an at-risk patient's informed choice is lacking, or an authorized proxy unavailable, "the physician must act in the best interest of the patient."[71] Acting humanely and with informed consent, a physician undertakes what is "medically necessary to alleviate severe pain, or cease or limit treatment to permit a terminally ill patient whose death is imminent to die" yet he should not follow a course of action that intentionally causes death.[72]

In making a decision whether the administration of potentially life-prolonging medical treatment (i.e., "medication and artificially or technologically supplied respiration, nutrition or hydration") comports with the incompetent patient's best interests, the physician is required to make a determination of what possibility exists for extending life under both humane and comfortable conditions. He is, furthermore, required to ascertain the patient's previously expressed wishes and the familial attitudes of others who have custodial responsibility for the patient.[73]

> Even if death is not imminent but a patient's coma is beyond doubt irreversible and there are adequate safeguards to confirm the accuracy of the diagnosis and with the concurrence of those who have responsibility for the care of the patient, it is not unethical to discontinue all means of life prolonging medical treatment. . . . In treating a terminally ill or irreversibly comatose patient, the physician should determine whether the benefits of treatment outweigh its burdens. At all times, the dignity of the patient should be maintained.[74]

Past Practices

At a Yale-New Haven Hospital symposium on "Ethical Issues in Health Care" in June, 1982, Dr. Paul B. Besson, the Editor of the Journal of the American Geriatrics Society, cautioned that there was a growing tendency in hospitals throughout the country to place "no-code" order on the hospital charts of a growing number of elderly patients.[75] Several years before Dr. Besson revealed his findings, a study of the records of nine convalescent centers (i.e., nursing and retirement homes) approved by the Federal medicare program in Seattle, Washington, and of the one thousand, two hundred and fifty-six persons admitted to these facilities in 1973 for a two-year period there were revealed some rather startling statistics.[76]

Over the period of the study, one hundred and ninety patients became febrile in that they developed a high or continuing fever at some time or had an impairment of their central nervous system (e.g., stroke, aphasia, paralysis, senility, dementia, chronic or organic brain syndrome and cerebral atheroarteriosclerosis). Active treatment—or the use of antibiotics or hospitalization or both—was ordered for but one hundred and nine patients. No such treatment was ordered or administered for eighty-one patients, or more than forty percent. Of those treated, nine percent died; and of those untreated, fifty-nine percent died. The authors of the study conclude that this obvious pattern of non-treatment suggests strongly that the physicians and nurses at these medical facilities studied did not intend to treat their patients actively when high mortality was expected.[77] It was determined that the lives of the untreated patients could have been prolonged for a short time if antibiotics had been administered or hospitalization followed.[78] The general conclusions of this study regarding the selective non-treatment of terminally ill, complements other surveys of health professionals favorably disposed to withdrawing or withholding life-prolonging treatment—with as many as thirty percent favoring euthanasia under certain prescribed conditions.[79]

In 1979, the Veterans Administration—which administers the largest hospital system in the nation with 1.2 million annual patient admissions—prohibited "no-code" or "do not resuscitate" orders being entered in a patient's medical chart.[80] In late August 1983, the Administration promulgated a new policy that, by recognizing a patient's right to die, allows "no-code" decisions to be written in a patient's chart.[81] Decisions of this nature must be made in turn by a senior physician with the permission of the at-risk patient. When the patient is not adjudged legally competent to make the decision, the consent of the family is necessary before it may be entered on the hospital records.[82] While the policy prohibits the use of a no-code order in those cases where a patient requests "voluntary euthanasia," and forbids physicians to "take any affirmative steps to 'hasten the patient on his/her way,'" in actuality what is seen here is a validation of a policy of passive euthanasia or letting die.[83] Application of the 1979 Veterans Administration Policy meant, simply, that if a physician had decided to respect the request or right of a patient to forego futile life-saving therapy, this decision could not be entered formally in the patient's hospital chart. Accordingly, in cases where such a patient suffered cardiac arrest and his understanding physician was not on duty, resuscitation would normally be undertaken against his wishes.

The new AMA policy incorporates an obvious quality of life standard of evaluation and it does so by utilizing the best interests of the patient test and mandating a cost-benefit analysis that in turn admixes principles of salvageability or *triage*.[84] Under basic social justice demands each individual should be given an opportunity to maximize his individual potential, a point is often reached where maintenance of an individual defies all concepts of not only social justice, but basic humanitarianism. When an individual's medical condition is such that it represents a negation of any "truly human" qualities or "relational-potential," then the best and most equitable form of treatment should be arguably no treatment at all.[85] In the final analysis, then, common sense and common decency should be the touchstones for decision making.

These policies of the American Medical Association[86] and the Veterans Administration[87] regarding the prolongation of medical treatment or what could be recognized as the right to die humanely and with dignity, coupled with the public medical record of actual occurrences of selective non-treatment of terminally ill[88], bear witness to the fact that intelligent health care providers are exercising common sense, common decency, love and compassion in their actions.[89] They are not bridled by complicated and obtuse distinctions between ordinary and extraordinary treatment standards, acts of commission and omission and a plethora of philosophical concerns over slippery slopes. Rather, they act courageously and forthrightly and are motivated by the age-old command to do no harm and thereby serve the best interests of their patients.[90]

Other Professional Postures

In 1983, The President's Commission for the Study of Ethical Problems in Medicine and Biomedical and Behavioral Research concluded that artificial feeding should be regarded as a treatment decision and not mandated except when the benefits of its use outweigh the burdens.[91] And, as mentioned previously, the American Medical Association's Council on Ethical and Judicial Affairs announced its conclusion in 1986 that all means of life-prolonging *treatment*—that included food as well as water—could be withdrawn from patients in an irreversible state or those in a terminal condition.[92]

The position of the Roman Catholic Church on the use of nutrition and fluids and the operative standard it follows where this issue is raised is that under some exceptional circumstances the means of providing nourishment may be such that it should not be regarded as obligatory owing to the ineffective or burdensome nature of the act, itself.[93] Thus, the withholding of nutrition and hydration does not have as its purpose the hastening of death—but rather the cessation of a life from which the patient can derive no benefit because of his futile or terminal condition.[94] With but one exception, the prominent Catholic theologians are of one mind: nutrition and fluids need not always "be provided to all patients, including the terminally ill."[95]

Even though a judicially determined order to withdraw life-sustaining treatment would, as a consequence of these three major policy clarifications, contain no affront if any form whatsoever to the integrity of the corporate hospital wherein the terminal patient might be or to the particular medical community treating him there, it may nonetheless be viewed by some health providers as an intolerable compromise or invasion of their own personal professional rights as physicians and nurses to use their skills in an actual effort to promote death.[96] In cases of this nature where this attitude exists, the only option should be for the dying patient to be transferred to another hospital willing to cease all artificial life supports and co-ordinate as dignified a death as possible.[97] When transfers are not feasible because of costs and/or of unavailable beds in other hospitals just for "dying," the issue becomes whether the care of a dying patient can be undertaken at home. Because of an unmistakable perception of pain, due to the marked change of appearance with a patient who is being withdrawn from fluids and nutrition, coping with at-home care can be difficult to manage or even sustained.[98] Thus it is seen that what might be thought of initially as a rather simple decision to withdraw treatment—and one to be respected—in reality, the decision is a very complex one that affects more than the dying patient and one not easily implemented.

An artful act of self-deception has been used in the past to deal with this issue and continues being used today.[99] Namely, intravenous feeding of a critically ill patient is continued—but at a diminished rate that, over time, will result in dehydration. Thus, both the gesture, and the equally important *symbol* of feeding is maintained, but at a rate that will not really sustain the patient's life for any period of time. Considered a "compromise" by those who wish desperately to hold to symbolic acts yet show some modicum of respect for the patient's direct wishes or perceived needs under a substituted judgment test or best interests to cease such treatment, this procedure is but a blatant act of self-deception,

... because an agent can carry it out only by failing to acknowledge that the patient will become malnourished and dehydrated while the IV line maintains the fiction and expresses the symbol of feeding. Otherwise the agent would have to take responsibility for the outcome. . . . [100]

The central question confronting the courts in regard to this issue is, "whether the corporate hospital should be required to provide services for its patients that the profession deems ethical and the courts hold to be lawful."[101] The modern hospital must be recognized, institutionally, as a center where whatever standard of care and treatment can be provided and relief of pain sought in the last rite of passage.[102]

Probably the overriding purpose of health law is to support medical and nursing care where the patient's wishes and best interests coincide. The coincidence of autonomy and appropriate health care is very clearly present when a competent judgment or substitute judgment is made, allowing a patient to spend his or her final brief moments of life in the health care setting that has been humanely treating and caring for the patient.[103]

When conscious awareness is lost and not capable of being re-established and all aspects of comfortable existence are removed as well, actions that omit nourishment by tubes, and not subterfuges for euthanasia, are but merely good medicine.[104]

The Hastings Center Guidelines

In issuing its Guidelines on *The Termination of Life Sustaining Treatment and the Care of the Dying,* in 1987, the prestigious Hastings Center of New York sought to set a new tone of acceptance and understanding of this area of concern. Consistent with the newly enacted Do Not Resuscitate Order Legislation in New York state,[105] the Guidelines structure an ethical framework for analyzing problem cases involving long-term life-supporting technology, ventilators and dialysis,[106] emergency interventions (e.g., cardiopulmonary resuscitation),[107] nutrition and hydration of terminal patients,[108] antibiotics and other life-sustaining medication,[109] and palliative care and pain relief.[110]

Central to any efforts of problem-solving here is an understanding, and thus an application, of four central values: 1) that the goal of medicine is always to promote the patient's well being or welfare; 2) a recognition of patient autonomy or self-determination that demands recognition of the right of the patient to determine the nature of his own medical care; 3) a realization that the integrity of health care professionals must be guaranteed by thus recognizing the stringent ethical obligations which physicians, nurses and other health care providers have to their patients; and 4) a need to realize the importance of the value of justice or equity in critical decisions of termination of treatment —or, in other words, the individual patient's right of access to an adequate level of health care as well as to the distribution of available health care resources.[111]

Of equal importance as a value in decision making of this nature, was the issue of costworthiness. It was determined quite directly that treatment that is wasteful, useless or harmful is simply not costworthy.[112] More specifically, it was found that:

> An ethic that aims to provide costworthy care cannot assume that any medical intervention that offers some benefit, no matter how marginal, should be provided regardless of its cost to others. Such an ethic must ask whether treatment that is marginally beneficial is costworthy in light of some satisfactory balance between benefit to the individual patient and alternative uses of these resources.[113]

These policy statements will be of indispensable value to health care professionals and other decision makers who are called upon to make the ultimate treatment decisions here. These policies should also be of considerable value to the legislatures who must act responsibly in designing frameworks, hopefully along the lines of the New York Do Not Resuscitate model, and to the courts when they are called upon to interpret legislation of this design.

Age-Based Rationing of Health Care

The director of the Hastings Center, Dr. Daniel Callahan, authored a controversial book in 1987 entitled, SETTING LIMITS: MEDICAL GOALS IN AN AGING SOCIETY, wherein he introduces the principle of age-based rationing[114] and argues persuasively that a national policy be introduced and implemented that prohibits the development or application of medical technologies to the old that are designed or likely "to produce only chronic illness and a short life, increase the present burden of chronic illness," or extend the lives of the elderly yet "offer no significant improvement in the quality of life."[115] The social policy which he calls for would—thus—limit life-extending treatment for the aged and could be implemented—additionally—by a simple denial of medicare benefits to various elderly groups.[116] To aid in determining these groups, various classifications are structured, based upon quality of life standards, designed as such to approach a determination of when morally appropriate care can be withheld.[117]

The underlying tenet of the framework is that if no genuine benefit is conferred upon the patient by the medical assistance that is questioned, and there is no meaningful life present, no life-prolonging actions should be undertaken.[118] Accordingly, if medical treatment can be stopped morally, food that is artificially provided as well as water can and should be stopped.[119] This later recognition is—as has been seen—the most difficult to accept or "sell" because it goes against the great moral tradition of meeting a societal "duty" to feed the hungry and provide water to the thirsty.[120]

I find Dr. Callahan's arguments to be very persuasive indeed. But, I find a strong inconsistency between the broad policy which he advocates for closing the limits of open-ended health care for the elderly by age-based rationing and his refusal to accept the rights of self-determination of the elderly through the legalization of assisted suicide or euthanasia.

Fearing such a policy "would serve as a threatening symbol of [the] devaluation of old age," Callahan expresses his fear that there "might be" a significant number of elderly drawn to this newly-approved situation because they would interpret the action or its legalized condonation "as a societal concession to the view that old age can have no meaning and significance if accompanied by decline, pain and despair."[121] It would approach an official recognition, "that pain is not to be endured, that community cannot be found for many of the old, and that a life not marked by good health, by hope and vitality, is not a life worth living."[122] To base a denial of full rights of self-determination for the elderly on fears of what "might happen" demeans the whole value of autonomy and constricts its application to only "approved" or presently "legitimate" purposes. It is the *individual*—regardless of age or infirmity—who should make the final determinations about his health care or medical needs. What official state policy is promoted by maintaining one in a state of "endured" pain? Are community values preserved by condoning a continuation of such states of human existence? I think not.

Handicapped Newborns

The Final Rule of the Department of Health and Human Services promulgated on April 15, 1985, entitled, "Child Abuse and Neglect Prevention and Treatment Program," is an effort to formulate a specific set of regulations regarding the medical treatment of severely handicapped newborns in state hospitals that receive federal grant assistance.[123] The withholding of medically indicated treatment—that includes "appropriate nutrition, hydration and medication"—is to provide all infants without exception, thereby leaving little latitude for medical judgment regarding their advisability. The three circumstances where treatment is not required are when the infant is either chronically and irreversibly comatose, "the treatment would merely prolong dying" and "not be effective in ameliorating or correcting all of the infant's life-threatening conditions, or otherwise be futile in terms of the survival of the infant and the treatment itself under such circumstances would be inhumane."[124]

Even though severely handicapped infants are unable to express preferences regarding a continuation or discontinuation of their lives, their incapacity should not mandate a course of medical therapy designed toward some degree of salvageability even though these actions prolong "life" (or, at least a semblance of it) at the cost of significant suffering.[125] "Where treatment has a high probability of causing significant pain and suffering and a low probability of preserving a life valuable to the patient, should we not permit a decision to withhold it?"[126]

The question to be raised in light of this government policy for handicapped newborns is whether a standard of aggressive treatment should in fact be implemented and thereby enforced for *all* incapacitated (e.g., incompetent) patients unless shown that death would occur in the near future or, alternatively, the patient is irreversibly comatose?[127]

> Is it always in the best interest of the elderly senile patient with advanced cancer to receive chemotherapy or radiation therapy until he is highly unlikely to survive beyond the near future? Should the severely debilitated (but not comatose) stroke victim be resuscitated an indefinite number of times until respiration cannot be restored by any means? There comes a point at which further prolongation of one's life simply does not make up for the burden of continued aggressive treatment, especially if the quality of life prolonged is diminished by suffering and incapacity. If it would be cruel to prolong the life of adult patients under these circumstances, then it must also be cruel to prolong the life of handicapped infants under comparable circumstances.[128]

Although inhumane or cruel treatment is one serious consideration, the other very practical one is an economic one, namely the need to find health care resources to meet the needs of those receiving life-prolonging treatments. Cost-benefit analysis becomes a valid consideration in rationing scarce medical resources.[129]

The distinction drawn between defective newborns and critically ill adults is most alarming. Somehow emotions and feelings run much higher and are made within a vortex of emotionalism when they are concerned with infants as opposed to adults and the elderly. Perhaps this is in part due to the fact that aspirations (hopes) are higher for the young than the old. In any event, decisions to withdraw or withhold treatment for both groups should be made when a cost-benefit analysis reveals the fact that costs of treatment outweigh the long-run benefits and best interests of the patient and are thus unreasonable.[130]

THE LEGAL PERSPECTIVE

A Right to Refuse Treatment?

The preservation or sanctity of life was and still is an important state interest in the common law; for common law has always held life is sacred and, thus, prohibited a person from either committing suicide or permitting his own destruction.[131] This general prohibition was equally applicable to those who were hopelessly ill as to those in good health.[132] A number or early cases likened a patient's refusal of life saving treatment to suicide and—accordingly—the state's interests in preserving the sanctity of life weighed against a patient's right to die with dignity.[133] More recent cases have tended to ignore the suicide analogy,[134] and some have failed to mention the state's interest in the sanctity of life at all.[135] The analogy to suicide is wholly inappropriate; for suicide is an act which has normally signified in the popular perception that life is worthless, while the decision to decline life saving medical measures is a choice involving death that does not express a realization that life is worthless. Indeed, to decline treatment does not imply a rejection of life any more than other behaviour which involves high risks to life and health. Similarly, the right to decline treatment does not imply a right to commit suicide.[136]

In addition to the state interest in the sanctity of life, it also—as a corollary—has a basic interest in preserving life, preventing suicide as mentioned, protecting incompetents and third party defendants as well as the preservation of the medical profession's integrity.[137] Thus, in validating or invalidating a right to die by refusing sustaining medical treatment, the courts will balance the individual rights of self-determination or autonomy against these state interests in forbidding a refusal of treatment. The nuances of this balancing test must—of necessity—tie to the facts of each case, for no unyielding *a priori* standard can be set and applied in an equally unyielding manner. Common sense and reasonable judgments are all that can be expected or actually made in tragic cases of this nature.[138]

The most significant state interest here is the preservation of life and what is, indeed, determined to be life is crucial to the assertion or maintenance by the state of its interest. The state will always act to prevent "irrational self-destruction."[139] The central question becomes, then, are there appropriately structured guidelines available to test the very rationality of decision making? What may seem reasonable to a legally competent but suffering patient may seem irrational to his attending physician. Sadly, what is seen—then—is that the determination of a patient's right to die is tied essentially to a judgment call.

Case precedent does, however, recognize that if compelled treatment will be brief and painful or extend life only as a consequence of great bodily intrusion, the "rationality" of original decision making by the patient will be given greater presumptive validity and—at the same time—the state interest in preserving life will be minimized.[140] Contrariwise, it could be maintained that a right to life exists where medical treatment preserves life, itself, rather than merely seeks to prolong it,[141] produces little, if any, pain and suffering, and constitutes no significant bodily intrusion.[142]

For the terminally ill patient, the qualitative value of sustained life should not be an issue of great moment; rather, it should be merely conceded that the dying processes should not be prolonged unduly.[143] For the non-terminal but chronically ill, retarded, debilitated or comatose patient, the state interest in preserving life is maintained if for no other reason than to protect such individuals from being eliminated, either by themselves when suffering from depression or under the direction of physicians who need hospital bed-space or families who can no longer bear the social and economic costs of maintaining their lives.[144]

Of course, such valid tests as "the best interest of the patient," and "the substituted judgment test" allow a court to inquire into the lengths to which state action should be allowed to force a continuation of life in a terminal state. The length of one's life expectancy before it becomes diagnosed affirmatively as *terminal* is a vexatious issue. Would an individual suffering from AIDS with an expected minimum of six years to live be recognized as non-terminal and, as such, be forced to live on by the state?[145] It has been suggested that the closer one's "life expectancy is to zero, the more the condition becomes 'terminal' and the patient's interests" more determinative.[146]

While there is thought to be a well-structured right of every competent person to refuse medical treatment based on any reason of his choice, a co-ordinate right to avoid being declared incompetent as a consequence of that basic refusal is only now beginning to be recognized.[147] Yet, thoughts aside, the United States Supreme Court has not made a definitive ruling that guarantees a constitutional right of an individual to forego a modality of medical treatment calculated to save his life.[148] Thus, care must be taken to recognize and deal separately with the related issues of whether other individuals are empowered to determine when and if life supports are not necessary in order to maintain continued existence.[149] Several prominent state jurisdictions have litigated the issue of the right of competents to refuse treatment and concluded such a qualified right does exist.[150]

The validation of a qualified right to die[151]—when made—is derived from several theories: the common law "right to bodily integrity,"[152] a so-called pneumbra "right of privacy" found by some courts in the Constitution,[153] the first amendment right of "free exercise of religion,"[154] and, to a growing extent, in state natural death legislation.[155] The right to refuse medical treatment and thus die has been recognized as but a "newly created constitutional right of personal autonomy."[156] There would seem to be a growing notion that a refusal of treatment decision should be as informed as the initiating consent to it;[157] and—set within the context of a critically ill person's decision making background—the doctrine of informed refusal is, indeed, an inherent part of the doctrine of informed consent.[158]

A Detailed Analysis of Leading Case Precedents

Surely, almost every week in some city, in some state, a scenario is being scripted that involves either a competent individual or one lacking in capacity because of infancy, mental incompetence or unconsciousness who is afflicted with an irreversible health condition that classifies him as terminal who wishes not to prolong his life. Some of these cases are reported by the local news, others in lower courts without official published records; but more and more wend their ways to appellate tribunals. It is neither the intention nor the purpose of this book to survey and then analyze cases. Rather, discussion of a number of the early and new paradigmatic "landmarks" is in order to place the ethical, philosophical, theological, medical and legal issues in a practical or working context.

The Precedental Core

In 1976, the New Jersey Supreme Court in the case of *In re Quinlan*,[159] while never referring specifically to a right to die, nonetheless implicitly —by analysis—determined that under particular circumstances, i.e., in the case of a terminal affliction that offers no hope of reversal, one—in effect—has a *right* to die. As such, *Quinlan* became the first major judicial decision approving the discontinuation of life-supporting treatments.[160]

Recognizing the past precedent of disallowing consent by the patient or third party as a defense to criminal liability, the court found other reasons to conclude an assessment of criminal liability would not be imposed under the facts of this case.[161] Specifically, since the disconnection of Ms. Quinlan's respirator would be a *natural* result of her affliction and thus not the criminal agency of the person, himself, who actually disconnected the respirator; and, furthermore, because the court tied its decision to the free exercise of Ms. Quinlan's right of privacy, the criminal law could not be utilized to punish the exercise of this constitutionally recognized right. This constitutional recognition—growing out of the holding in *Griswold v. Connecticut*,[162] thereby served as a protection or grant of immunity to individuals here—the physicians—who effectuate the exercise of the privacy right.[163]

Ms. Quinlan's father—supported unanimously by the family—was given the authority to withdraw the respirator that all medical experts agreed was keeping her alive. But, tragically, she remained alive for some nine years after she was removed from the respirator. Even though this withdrawal of artificial respiration occurred, it is interesting to note that her father never sought judicial permission to withdraw nutrition and hydration from her—acts in and of themselves that could be recognized as extraordinary given the prognosis of her recovery.[164]

One year after *Quinlan* in 1977, came a controversial decision by the Massachusetts Supreme Judicial Court, *Superintendent of Belchertown State School v. Saikewicz*.[165] There it was held that before Joseph Saikewicz, a sixty-seven-year-old patient at a state mental health facility, profoundly retarded with an I.Q. of 10, a mental age of two-and-a-half years old with an inability to communicate verbally and suffering from an incurable form of leukemia, could decline an extraordinary course of treatment (e.g., chemotherapy) that would sustain his life (and possibly present a chance of a two-to-thirteen month remission) but bring complicated and serious painful side effects,[166] a probate court would first determine whether he, as an incompetent, had properly exercised his right to refuse treatment guaranteed him by the fourteenth amendment's right of privacy.[167]

Although criticized by the medical profession as an offensive and unwarranted intrusion into the practice of medicine and the confidentiality of the doctor-patient relationship,[168] the court reasoned that it had no other recourse than to intervene and, utilizing the doctrine of substituted judgment, determine whether Mr. Saikewicz would have wished the invasive medical treatment,[169] and his best interests would in fact be served by such a course of action.[170] The court struggled with its responsibility to preserve life yet maintain the personal autonomy of all citizens and guarantee that their best interests were protected if not advanced in all circumstances.[171] It also inherently utilized a cost-benefit analysis in applying the primary doctrine of substituted judgment,[172] evaluating the potential for short-term benefits from the chemotherapy versus the long term pain, discomfort and disorientation that would follow.[173] The value of the *potential* remission was not adjudged significant enough to merit the chemotherapy treatment.[174]

Within a year, a new Massachusetts case was litigated that departed from *Saikewicz*.[175] In this case, *In re Dinnerstein*,[176] the Massachusetts Court of Appeal was presented with a case of first impression: namely the issuance of an order not to resuscitate (ONTR). Its holding was that an attending family physician may, acting with family consent or agreement and without prior approval from a probate court, issue an ONTR in the event of respiratory failure or cardiac arrest for a patient who is incompetent and terminally ill.[177]

Recognizing that the case presented questions directly within the competence of the medical profession regarding those effects thought to ease the death of an irreversibly terminally ill patient in light of her past medical history and consistent with her family's wishes, the court found no reason to apply the doctrine of substituted judgment.[178] Here, Shirley Dinnerstein was a sixty-seven-year-old widow, in the advanced stages of Alzheimer's disease, with a coronary condition who suffered a stroke — brain death not being an issue. Her adult son and daughter together with her physician sought declaratory relief in order to determine whether her attending physician could lawfully enter a "no code" order if she suffered cardiopulmonary arrest. *Dinnerstein,* unlike *Saikewicz,* could not be construed as a "right to treatment" case, simply because of the fact that there was no course of treatment that would improve significantly and in the long run her degenerative condition.

The difference in *Dinnerstein* and *Saikewicz* then, is not as startling as first might have appeared; for the two Massachusetts courts are merely making a valid and thoughtful distinction between a patient who will at some time in the near future die from one who is in the current process of dying. The significance of this distinction was stated and elaborated upon by the Massachusetts Supreme Judicial Court in its case of *In re Spring,*[179] handed down two years later.

In Spring, the facts revealed that Earle N. Spring, a seventy-seven-year-old man suffering from advanced senility and end-stage kidney disease, was being heavily sedated three times a week (in order to abate his resistance) to receive five hour hemodialysis treatments and thereby have his life sustained. Both his wife of some fifty-five years and his only son requested his treatment be stopped; but his physicians refused to comply.[180] Thereupon, a judgment from the probate court was sought by Mrs. Spring and her son (who had become his temporary legal guardian in January, 1979) for an order directing that the life-sustaining treatment be ceased.[181] In May, 1979, the probate court held an evidentiary hearing and received the report of the guardian *ad litem* whom it had appointed for Earle Spring; and ruled consequently that all treatment decisions were to be made by Mrs. Spring and her son *and* the attending physician. The guardian *ad litem* appealed and, granting the motion, the probate court stayed its own judgment.[182]

On appeal, the *Spring* court chose to draw a distinction between a patient for whom further treatment would be of no value and one for whom additional treatment would be a genuine alternative. Although the court concluded that death was indeed inevitable for Mr. Spring, it acknowledged the remote possibility that he "might regain competence, experience lucid intervals, or even be able to express a 'sensible opinion' as to his desire,"[183] and thus force the court to modify its order.[184] After affirming *Saikewicz*, the court ordered no further use of life-prolonging treatment and went further to hold that the probate court, and it alone, not Mr. Spring's wife or his son or attending physician, was the proper party to determine the extent to which the substituted judgment standard would be applied.[185] Here, it was found the standard of substituted judgment had, indeed, been properly applied and met.[186]

In New York, the judicial temperament was less understanding and more conservative in its analysis of decisions to forego treatment than in Massachusetts. For, with two decisions, *In re Eichner*[187] and *In re Storar*[188] it was held that it was unnecessary to determine whether the right to refuse treatment was an inherent element in the fourteenth amendment's right to privacy because common law principles supported its recognition;[189] that the doctrine of substituted judgment was not a point of contention because clear and convincing evidence would always be required of an individual's decision to initiate or discontinue treatment before he became incompetent in order for a court to sanction its operation;[190] and that, furthermore, the doctrine of substituted judgment as applied in *Saikewicz* under surprisingly similar facts here in *Storar* was an unrealistic application and that life-prolonging treatment of a terminally ill incompetent cancer victim could not be withdrawn.[191]

In *Eichner*, an eighty-three-year-old member of the Roman Catholic Society of Mary, Brother Fox, went in to cardiac arrest during a routine hernia operation. He lost oxygen for but a few moments and was placed, while in a state of coma, on a respirator. Substantial brain damage as a consequence of these events determined that he would have no reasonable chance of making any type of recovery. When a close friend, Father Philip Eichner, directed that the respirator be removed, the hospital refused and this present action was initiated.[192] The Appellate Division of the Supreme Court held that the right to refuse treatment was an inherent guarantee found within the Common Law and protected, additionally, by the fourteenth amendment's right to privacy and that this right could, through application of the doctrine of substituted judgment, be exercised under the facts of the instant case. Heavy reliance was placed upon the *Saikewicz* and *Spring* Massachusetts precedents.[193] The New York Court of Appeal, for the large part, rejected much of the appellate court's analysis and skirted the major problem by finding that Brother Fox had, himself, before he ever became incompetent, given compelling proof of his views on the issue by relating to Father Eichner that he never wished to be maintained on artificial life supports.[194]

In the companion case of *In re Storar*,[195] a fifty-two-year-old retarded man, John Storar, was afflicted with terminal bladder cancer causing him to lose blood regularly and thus be subjected to blood transfusions in order to replace that which he lost. His mother and guardian sought to have the transfusions discontinued—even though the son had more energy after them and was able to resume his "normal" routine.[196] Finding that because of his infant mentality it would be totally unrealistic to ascertain his wishes about a continuation of potentially life-prolonging treatment if he were in fact competent, the court held that the artifice of substituted judgment could not be employed by an infant's parent or guardian to thereby deprive a child of life-saving treatment—especially since the transfusions were analogous to food.[197] Tragically, while being so quick to criticize and reject the validity or application of the doctrine of substituted judgment, the court chose to disregard the opportunity of developing a new framework for principled decision making and instead called upon a mandatory procedure to be forthcoming from the legislature.[198]

In the combined decision in *Barber v. Superior Court of Los Angeles County and Nejdl v. Superior Court of Los Angeles County* in 1983[199] the California Court of Appeal for the Second District for the first time, equated the discontinuation of an intravenous feeding with the removal of a respirator or any other medical intervention.[200] Each, it declared, was a medical treatment and, as such, was to be used only if it benefits the patient.[201] Thus, if the intervention merely sustains biological functions, it should not be regarded as a treatment—but, rather a useless gesture and one the physician is not obligated to follow.[202] What becomes especially significant here is the court's shift in its analysis from the more traditional emphasis of "ordinary v. extraordinary" means of treatment to a "proportionate-disproportionate" benefits standard[203] thereby transferring the emphasis from the multitude of medical techniques and processes involved to the *condition* of the patient if these mechanisms are started or retained.[204]

> Thus, even if a proposed course of treatment might be extremely painful or intrusive, it would still be proportionate treatment if the prognosis was for complete cure or significant improvement in the patient's condition. On the other hand, a treatment course which is only minimally painful or intrusive may nonetheless be considered

disproportionate to the potential benefits if the prognosis is virtually hopeless for any significant improvement in condition.[205]

Shortly after surgery for closure of an ileostomy, Clarence Herbert suffered a cardiopulmonary arrest, went into a coma and was placed on a respirator. After five days, the physicians determined his condition to be irreversible and so advised his wife and family. With permission from the wife being obtained, use of the respirator was discontinued. Tragically, Mr. Herbert continued, nevertheless, to live—however—still in a state of coma.[206] Thereupon, the doctors received written permission from Mrs. Herbert to terminate the administration of nutrition and hydration. Six days later, he died—but during those days he "received nursing care which preserved his dignity and provided a clean and hygienic environment."[207]

The issue confronting the court of appeal was whether the two attending physicians, Dr. Barber and Dr. Nejdl, should be held guilty of murder and conspiracy to commit murder.[208] The court, in reaching a conclusion that no charge of this nature would be sustained, chose to view the conduct of the physicians "as that of omission rather than affirmative action."[209]

> There is no criminal liability for failure to act unless there is a legal duty to act. . . . "[210] A physician has no duty to continue treatment, once it has proved to be ineffective. Although there may be a duty to provide life-sustaining machinery in the immediate aftermath of a cardiopulmonary arrest, there is no duty to continue its use once it has become futile in the opinion of qualified personnel.[211]
> . . . . No precise guidelines as to when or how these decisions should be made can be provided by this court since this determination is essentially a medical one to be made at a time and on the basis of facts which will be unique to each case.[212]

The *Barber-Nejdl* court stressed its position that judicial intervention was not required in cases of this nature, unless legislative direction so ordered. Indeed, a requirement of judicial intervention in all similar cases should be viewed as not only unnecessary, but unwise.[213] Agreeing that Mrs. Herbert was the proper surrogate decision maker for her husband and that his previous expressions of not wishing to "become another Karen Ann Quinlan" had been taken into full account regarding the ultimate decision here, the court determined in those cases where it was not possible to determine the choice the patient would have made, the surrogate should be guided in his decision making by the "patient's best interests."[214]

In April, 1984, seventy-year-old William Bartling was admitted to the Glendale Adventist Hospital in California for treatment of depression.[215] Suffering from emphysema, arteriosclerosis and an abdominal aneurysm, an examination revealed him to have a malignant lung tumor. During efforts to obtain a biopsy of the tumor, however, the lung collapsed and failed to reinflate; thus a tracheotomy was performed and Mr. Bartling placed on a respirator.[216] Requests made by Mr. Bartling and his wife to the physicians for the removal of the respirator were to no avail—so in June, 1984, an injunction was sought by Mr. Bartling to prohibit both the hospital and the physicians alike from administering further treatment as well as damages for treatment without his consent in violation of his state and constitutional rights and for not only breach of the fiduciary duty owed to him by the hospital and his treating physicians but also for intentional infliction of emotional distress and conspiracy.[217]

Mr. Bartling had executed a non-statutory "living will" signed by him with an X and properly witnessed stating his direction that should be placed in a situation of "extreme physical or mental disability" where there was no "reasonable expectation" of recovery, he wished to be allowed to die.[218] Additionally, he had had executed a declaration under the state Natural Death Act underscoring his wish to die with dignity and continue in the "intolerable" manner in which he was living as a consequence of his deteriorating health.[219] He also executed a durable power of attorney for health care with his wife wherein he directed her as his "attorney-in-fact" to honor his desire to end his "humiliating indignity" by refusing ventilator support.[220] Both Mr. Bartling and his wife—together with their daughter—signed a release from civil liability for the hospital and their physicians.[221] In spite of all of these measures, the physicians found Mr. Bartling's condition not terminal—in that he could live for a year if weaned from the respirator even though real doubts existed about the feasibility of this action and they questioned his ability to make a meaningful decision, although not questioning his legal competency. They also expressed concern about the ethics of disconnecting life support and the potential civil and criminal liability that might follow their actions.[222]

The court held that the right to disconnect a life-support mechanism was not limited to only comatose or terminally ill patients.[223] Grounded in a constitutional right of privacy as it emerges from the Fifth and Ninth Amendments, this right of the patient self-determination is to be regarded as "paramount to the interests of the patient's hospital and doctors" regarding their concern of professional ethical violations for disconnecting a life-support system.[224]

Disregarding the assertion that the state had a positive interest in protecting against suicide, the court held that the state's interest was in protecting only against "irrational self-destruction," and what was seen here was a,

> competent, rational decision to refuse treatment when death is inevitable and the treatment offers no hope or cure of preservation of life. There is no connection between the conduct here in issue and any State concerns to prevent suicide.[225]

The court held that no civil or criminal liability would attach to the act of disconnecting the life-sustaining equipment—this, consistent with Mr. Bartling's request; and, that, furthermore no advance judicial approval or intervention would be required here.[226] The fact that Mr. Bartling executed his declaration and in his supporting documents also attested to his wish to die with dignity was sufficient evidence that he was aware that he would die if disconnected from the ventilator.[227] Although finding that the California Natural Death Act applied only to a narrow number of individuals who were certified as terminally ill and that a directive under it was not the exclusive method of refusing treatment, the court chose not to set forth a defined structure for competent patients to follow in this regard.[228]

In 1979, Claire Conroy was eighty-four years of age and residing in a nursing home. She was ambulatory and although often confused, she was able to converse.[229] She was afflicted with arteriosclerotic heart disease, hypertension, diabetes and a gangerous leg and employed a urinary catheter and had no bowel control.[230] Between 1979 and 1983, these conditions became exacerbated and she was afflicted with severe organic brain syndrome.[231] A nasogastric tube was subsequently inserted that supplied her with nutrients and fluids. Her life expectancy with the tubal feeding was set at no more than a year; without it she was expected to die of dehydration within approximately a week's time.[232]

In 1983, Ms. Conroy's nephew sought judicial authorization for the removal of the nasogastric tube so that she might die.[233] While the trial agreed that when intelligence had been reduced permanently as here, with a corresponding array of medical difficulties that life had, indeed, become impossible, the tubal nourishment could be withdrawn even though the ensuing starvation might be painful in nature to Ms. Conroy.[234]

Although not disputing the contention of Ms. Conroy's nephew that if she had been competent she would have wished to be taken from her artificial (tubal) nourishment, the intermediate appellate court refused to sustain the order of the lower court.[235] Central to its reasoning was the fact that she appeared to be suffering no pain, and that she well might endure it if the tubal feeding were to stop;[236] and since she was neither in a terminal condition nor permanently comatose or in a chronic vegetative state; and thus not in a state of imminent death,[237] routine life supports such as nutrition could *not* be withdrawn because the state interest in preserving life supports such as nutrition could *not* be withdrawn because the state interest in preserving life simply outweighed Ms. Conroy's privacy intent.[238] Also of consideration was the fact that before a right of termination of life-sustaining treatment was recognized judicially, there would need to be shown that the patient would gain no medical benefit from the continuation of present treatment; and no conclusive evidence on this point was shown in Ms. Conroy's care.[239]

The New Jersey Supreme Court reversed the Appellate Division and held that even though Ms. Conroy had died (with the nasogastric tube in place) before the conclusion of the case, her death did not moot the case—this owing to the fact that the issues raised by it were of great moment and would likely be arising again; that a competent adult has a general right to refuse life-sustaining medical treatment (here, nutrients) and does not because of subsequent incompetency, lose it; if certain procedures are followed in certain defined sets of circumstance, a surrogate decision maker may—acting on behalf of the incompetent—withdraw life-sustaining treatment.[240]

Behind this determination was a rather complex procedure that the court requires to be followed before a decision to terminate treatment (such as artificial feeding) could be withdrawn from a dying patient. Indeed, for elderly incompetent nursing home residents who "will probably die within approximately one year even with treatment" treatment could be withheld if three conditions were met: 1.) It was clear that the particular patient would have refused treatment under the present circumstances (or the subjective test);[241] 2.) There is some indication of the patient's wishes—even though he has not "unequivocally expressed" his desires before becoming incompetent—and the course of treatment "would only prolong suffering" (the limited-objective test);[242] and 3.) When there is no evidence of any nature regarding the patient's wishes but the treatment "clearly and markedly outweighs the benefits the patient derives from life" (the pure objective test).[243]

Under the implementing procedures set forth by the court, in the case of an incompetent patient, a judicial determination must be made that the incompetent is incompetent to make the decision himself regarding the withholding or withdrawing of life-sustaining medical treatment. If no guardian has heretofore been appointed, the court will do so after this determination. Even if previously adjudicated as incompetent, a specific determination must be made whether the patient can make the *present* decision concerning medical treatment. If a guardian has already been appointed for the patient, the judicial inquiry must be directed to the suitability of the guardian, himself, to make this decision.[244]

The guardian—or other person—who holds the opinion that the actions of withholding or withdrawing would either effectuate the patient's wishes *or* meet either the second or third tests and, thus, be in his "best interests," must thereupon notify the office of the State Ombudsman of the action that is contemplated presently. Similarly, for any person who considers the contemplated action would be an abuse to the at-risk patient, contact with the Ombudsman may be obtained. Upon notification of a possible abuse, the Ombudsman is required to investigate it and report the matter to the Commissioner of Human Services and other concerned administrative officials.[245]

The attending physician and nurses are required to furnish evidence concerning the patient's condition; and two other doctors, unaffiliated with the case or the institution where the patient is being maintained should be appointed to confirm both the condition of the patient and his prognosis. If the two physicians present the necessary medical foundation, the guardian may then—with the concurrence of the attending physician and the Ombudsman—proceed to either withhold or withdraw life-sustaining medical treatment if a good faith belief is held, based upon the medical evidence as well as any additional evidence of the wishes of the patient, that it is clear that at least one of the three tests is met. In the case of the use of the limited-objective test, the patient's next of kin must also concur.[246] Because of the complexity of the tests and their implementing procedure, it is very difficult to imagine a situation developing where treatment would be withheld or withdrawn under the *Brophy* structure.[247]

On February 26, 1986, a New Jersey State Superior Court Judge ruled that Nancy Ellen Jobes—a thirty-year-old married woman, who had been unconscious since April, 1980—had a right of self-determination to have a feeding jejunostomy tube, that was surgically implanted in her small intestine that received liquid nutrition and water from a continuous drip regulated by a pump, removed (by a physician).[248] This action was maintained for removal of her feeding system by Mrs. Jobes's husband. The Lincoln Park Nursing Home, where Mrs. Jobes was a patient, opposed the action and sought its own appointment as a "life advocate" who would "fight for the life" of Mrs. Jobes.[249]

In disallowing the claim of the nursing home for an appointment as a guardian *ad litem,* the court observed that

> . . . it is not the function of the guardian *ad litem* in these life-support cases to argue for continuation of the incompetent ward's life in each and every case. Such a view misconceives the time-honored obligation of the guardian *ad litem* to act in the *best interests* of the ward.[250]

Explaining that a policy that mandated extraordinary life-supporting measures to be maintained in all cases involving terminal care, would violate an individual's constitutional and common law right of privacy, the court concluded that both the competent and the incompetent possess the *same* right of self-determination in matters of this nature.[251]

In a 6-1 decision, delivered June 24, 1987, the New Jersey Supreme Court found that the trial court had properly determined that there was "clear and convincing" evidence that Mrs. Jobes was in a persistent vegetative state—this, in spite of the fact that two nursing home examining physicians (neurologists) maintained she fell slightly outside the definition of being in this state.[252] Finding further that the situation in which Nancy Jobes was in was directly analogous to that of Karen Quinlan's case, the High Court held that nutrition and hydration were medical treatment issues and could be withheld or withdrawn on behalf of the afflicted patient.[253] Interestingly, on this point, the trial court's finding, that clear and convincing evidence had been adduced, was reversed—it being determined that Mrs. Jobes had not been sufficiently specific to be considered as "clear and convincing," but instead were statements that were "remote, general, spontaneous and made in casual circumstances."[254]

Even with this ruling, Justice Garibaldi—speaking for the majority Court—acknowledged tubal feeding could be ended if members of the Jobes family (spouse, parents, adult children or siblings or another relative who could be regarded as a part of the patient's nuclear family) exercise their best, substituted judgment regarding the wishes of "the motives and considerations that would control the patient's medical decisions."[255] If close and caring members of the patient's family are willing to make critical care decisions, no guardian need to be appointed and, thus, no judicial review of the decisions need be undertaken.[256] If the patient has no close family members, however, and has failed to establish—over the course of his active life—clear and convincing evidence of his wish to have a distant relative or friend make a surrogate medical decision of the nature required in cases of this nature, if he is incompetent, a guardian must be appointed.[257]

Even though Mrs. Jobes was in a nursing home, the court determined that the decision making process for surrogates "should be substantially the same regardless of where the patient is located."[258] The court proceeded to establish a set of guidelines that, if followed in good faith, would remove criminal or civil liability for the implementation of any surrogate decision to decline medical treatment.[259] Simple and straightforward, the guidelines do recognize that there are certain safeguards that exist within hospital settings that are not usually found in nursing homes.[260] Thus, for the patient under sixty years of age in a nursing home who is—accordingly—"non-elderly" and "non-hospitalized" but "in a persistent vegetative state, the surrogate decision maker who declines life-sustaining medical treatment must secure statements from at least two independent physicians that the patient is in a persistent vegetative state and that there is no reasonable possibility that the patient will ever recover."[261]

The New Jersey Supreme Court reversed the holding of the lower court that allowed the Lincoln Park Nursing Home to refuse to participate in the withdrawal of Mrs. Jobes's feeding tube.[262] The court reasoned that since the Jobes family had no reason to believe it was foregoing the right to select among various medical alternatives when Mrs. Jobes was placed in Lincoln Park and—furthermore—because it would be extremely burdensome to locate another nursing home facility that would accept her, to allow the Lincoln Park Home to discharge her would, in essence, frustrate her right of self-determination.[263]

This ruling is thought of as extending both *Quinlan*[264] and *Conroy*[265] in that while removal of a respirator may or may not cause death within the foreseeable future as with Ms. Quinlan's case, the withdrawal of artificial feeding and its recognition thereby as treatment, means that in most cases death will occur within one or two weeks.[266] And, in *Conroy,* the court—while recognizing artificial feeding was a medical procedure and potentially could be withdrawn from a dying patient—for incompetent nursing home residents, a complicated procedure was set forth making the whole matter exceedingly cumbersome.[267] With *Jobes,* the simple recognition of the right of self-determination and its co-ordinate right of withdrawal of *treatment* made the process neat and unencumbered.[268]

When, on November 1, 1983, Elizabeth Bouvia—a competent, college-educated, non-terminally ill county hospital patient applied to a court of law for permission to starve herself to death because her disabilities were such as to make her unable to take her own life,[269] never was it realized that her quest for enlightened self-determination would not be recognized until April 16, 1986.[270] Her first effort sought a prohibitory injunction against the Riverside General Hospital from administering any health care without her consent and, furthermore, by installing or inserting by any method an intravenous, nasogastric or gastrostomy tubation or tubing to sustain her.[271] The essence of her claim was that she had the right of personal autonomy or self-determination to decide when and how her life should end, and that there was a societal obligation to render her assistance in the execution of that right.[272] The defendants answered by alleging that she had no such statutory, constitutional, ethical or moral right to undertake this action and—alternatively—if she did have the right it could be overcome by compelling state interests.[273]

Since birth, Ms. Bouvia has suffered from severe cerebral palsy and as a quadriplegic has virtually no motor function in her limbs. She does have slight muscle control that allows her to operate an electric wheelchair. Voluntary control of her face, mouth and throat allows her to eat a normal diet fed to her and to converse. At this point in time, her cerebral palsy was not of a progressive nature.[274] The trial court judge found that Ms. Bouvia did have the right, under the unwritten right of privacy and self-determination found in the First, Fourth, Fifth and Fourteenth Amendments, to terminate her existence—but not while she was in a non-terminal condition with the assistance of society.[275] Therefore, petition for injunctive relief was denied; and the court, without any supporting authority, went on to admonish Ms. Bouvia that "there is hope in life" and that she could be a "symbol of hope" to others similarly situated.[276] It was thought that she could have from fifteen to twenty years of "life" left.[277]

Although recognizing her rationality and competency to make her decision,[278] the court concluded the allowance of such a request as was sought in equity would have "a profound effect on the medical staff, nurses and administration" of her treating hospital.[279] Furthermore, the motive behind the anticipated act, and the actual act itself, of starvation by Ms. Bouvia would constitute suicide and therefore run counter to the state's interest in preserving life and preventing the assistance of its being taken.[280] It has been submitted that Ms. Bouvia was discriminated by her handicap in that she was prevented from exercising an ability to achieve an act (e.g., starvation) and that an equally competent person who is not physically incapable can do without restriction.[281]

In the case of a young woman, such as Ms. Bouvia, who openly contemplates her suicide, surely reasonable efforts should be made in order to not only assess her competency but to dissuade her from self-destruction. The testing area is what happens after reasonable steps fail. Perhaps, after a waiting period of some six months where within this period psychiatric assessment and psychological counseling can be given, a re-evaluation of an initial request for starvation could be made.[282] Owing to the fact here that Ms. Bouvia had had previous hospitalization of several days in order to "change her mind," perhaps it is possible that further hospitalization and forced feeding would allow her to once again change her mind.[283] Although forced feeding of a competent adult raises serious issues of individual autonomy and integrity, efforts to persuade and *offer* oral nutrition should perhaps continue.[284] But beyond these actions set within a defined time frame, it would appear brutal and unconscionable to require more than this.[285]

By the time her appeal was decided, April 16, 1986, Ms. Bouvia—now twenty-eight years of age—had regrettably deteriorated to such an extent that her palsy and quadriplegia were now joined with a degenerative and very crippling type of arthritis. She was completely bed-ridden and—for the exception of slight head and facial movements—was physically helpless and dependent upon the care of others.[286] She must lie flat on her back for the remainder of her life, suffering pain continually. In addition to tubal liquid feeding, she has another tube attached permanently to her chest that injects her periodically with morphine in order to relieve some of her pain.[287] The court granted Ms. Bouvia's request for preliminary injunction and ordered directly that her nasogastric tube be removed and its further use be prohibited and, additionally, that its replacement or any such device like it could not be done without her request.

Noting the factual similarity of Ms. Bouvia's condition with William

Bartling,[288] and the similarity of issues here and in *Barber*,[289] the court declares a patient's right to refuse any medical treatment or medical service even though such may be termed nourishment and hydration and even if such actions precipitate a life-threatening condition.[290] Observing that Ms. Bouvia is neither comatose, vegetative or in a terminal condition—as she could well survive another fifteen or twenty years[291] —the court also took cognizance that the quality of that existence had in her view become hopeless, useless, unenjoyable and frustrating.[292]

The court determined that the right or refusal derives from not only the right of privacy protected by the state and federal constitutions, but by case precedent—*Bartling* and *Barber*, specifically—and the California Natural Death Act.[293] And, furthermore, that the decision to forego mechanical treatment is solely within her own province to determine.[294]

> It is not a medical decision for her physician to make. Neither is it a legal question whose soundness is to be resolved by lawyers or judges. It is not a conditional right subject to approval by ethics committees or courts of law. It is a moral and philosophical decision that, being a competent adult, is hers alone.[295]

Regarding motive, the court determined that if a right is recognized as existing, the motivation behind its exercise is of no consequence.[296] Thus, the right can be exercised without its approval by any other person. And, hence, in no way can the right to refuse treatment be characterized as suicide or an assistance of it.[297] Citing California case precedence to support its finds on this point,[298] the court observes that, traditionally, the means to effect or assist a suicide involved conduct that was affirmative in nature, proximate or direct—such as furnishing a gun or poison—or other type of instrumentality that would inflict an immediate "death producing injury." "Here all that is being considered is the presence of a doctor directing the exercise of a constitutional right."[299]

Prior to March 22, 1983, Paul Brophy had been a healthy and robust forty-nine-year-old emergency medical technician and fireman in Easton, Massachusetts. On the evening of the twenty-second, he suffered the rupture of an aneurysm at the apex of his basilar artery (although not considered brain dead).[300] He failed to regain consciousness and became vegetative—being kept alive by the maintenance of a surgically inserted device, or gastrostomy tube (G-tube) through which he received nutrition and hydration.[301] When the hospital where Mr. Brophy was a patient refused to respect the family decision to have the feeding tube removed or clamped, Mrs. Brophy sought legal redress.[302] The trial court, while acknowledging that—if competent—Mr. Brophy would decline the use of the G-tube, it nonetheless refused to permit removal—arguing that the state's interest in preserving life outweighed his right to choose his form of treatment.[303] Here, on expedited appeal, the Massachusetts High Court found, on the basis of the doctrine of substituted judgment, that the personal rights of self-determination and individual autonomy arising from the Common Law and the "unwritten and penumbral constitutional right to privacy" allowed him—through his surrogate decision maker, his wife—to refuse medical treatment;[304] and that this right was superior to that of the state interest in preserving life.[305]

Drawing upon past precedents,[306] the court concluded that when efforts to sustain life were demeaning or degrading to one's humanity, an individual had every right to avoid such circumstances.[307] The court acknowledged that while the distinction between ordinary and extraordinary care was a factor of some meritorious consideration here, its use should not be the primary factor in decision making.[308]

> ... to state that the maintenance of nutrition and hydration by the use of the existing G-tube is only ordinary is to ignore the total circumstances of Brophy's situation. He cannot swallow ... to be maintained by such artificial means over an extended period is not only intrusive but extraordinary.[309]

In response to the hospital's argument that it was not obligated by constitutional, statutory or common law rights to deny nutrition and hydration in order to facilitate Mr. Brophy's death, and that—furthermore—the moral and ethical principles of the medical profession forbade such practices, the High Court agreed with the conclusion of the probate court that this argument was sound.[310] The court found that neither the doctrine of informed consent, the Massachusetts Patients Right Statute "nor any other provision of law requires the hospital to cease hydration and nutrition upon request of the guardian."[311] Acknowledging that *Saikewicz*[312] and its "progeny" would not compel health care providers to undertake measures that would be regarded as contrary to their views of the nature and scope of their patient duties, the court concludes the right of a patient to refuse medical treatment "does not warrant such an unnecessary intrusion upon the hospital's ethical integrity in this case."[313] Thus, the solution to this quandry is to but order the Mount Sinai hospital where Mr. Brophy is a patient to "assist" in transferring him to a suitable facility where his primary wishes may be, through his guardian, effectuated.[314]

Since *Brophy* is the first written state supreme court opinion authorizing artificial, tubal feeding to be removed during the patient's present existence, it is to be viewed as quite significant. Particularly so because of its finding that a feeding tube may be intrusive and considered extraordinary treatment[315] and that when such a tube is accordingly removed from a persistently vegetative patient, the cause of death should be understood as the underlying condition preventing swallowing—not the removal of the tube.[316]

Brophy's significance goes even farther in that it re-enforces, if not legitimizes, a developing judicial trend that acknowledges the right of a patient to refuse artificial feeding as he would all other medical treatments;[317] that there is no valid moral distinction between withholding treatment and withdrawing treatment; a refusal of life-sustaining treatment is not synonymous with suicide—indeed, it is inapplicable;[318] and an incompetent patient's substituted judgment outweighs the state's interest in preserving life even though he is not diagnosed as terminal. In light of the anticipated far-reaching effect of this notable trend allowing a right of refusal for artificial feeding as other medical treatment, it may be expected that state legislature would be cautioned against enacting legislation that would seek to prohibit artificial feeding.[319]

The Aftermath

Quinlan, Saikewicz, Dinnerstein, Spring, Barber, Bartling, Conroy, Brophy, Jobes and *Bouvia* all point with unremitting clarity to the fact that more and more courts are respecting acts of enlightened self-determination by competent patients—or their surrogate decision makers—to withhold or withdraw life-sustaining medical treatments, even though by doing so death results.[320] Behind the extended judicial rhetoric of balancing individual privacy interests and rights of self-determination against countervailing state interests in preserving life, preventing suicide, safeguarding the integrity of the medical profession and protecting innocent third parties,[321] "is a highly predictable endpoint of judicial reasoning":[322] namely, that once it is clear or at least reasonably understood that one has chosen to end his life by refusing life-sustaining medical treatment, the appellate courts will respect and uphold this decision as within his common law right of autonomy or self-determination of the pneumbra right of privacy found within the Fourteenth Amendment to the Constitution.[323]

ENDNOTES

1. See Standards for Cardiopulomany Resuscitation (CPR) and Emergency Cardiac Care (ECC), 227 J.A.M.A. 837 (1974).

See generally, Evans & Brody, The Do-Not-Resuscitate Order in Teaching Hospitals, 253 J.A.M.A. 2236 (1985).

2. Id.

3. Id.

See, Miller, Death with Dignity and the Right to Die: Sometimes Doctors Have a Duty to Hasten Death, 13 J. MED. ETHICS 81 (1987).

4. P. RAMSEY, THE PATIENT AS PERSON 239–246 (1970).

See also, Smith, Death Be Not Proud: Medical, Ethical and Legal Dilemmas in Resource Allocation, 3 J. CONTEMP. HEALTH L. & POL'Y 47 (1987).

5. Capron, Legal and Ethical Problems in Decisions for Death, 14 LAW, MED. & HEALTH CARE 141 (1986).

6. Id.

7. Id.

8. Id.

9. See generally, Comment, A Structural Analysis of the Physician-Patient Relationship in No-Code Decisionmaking, 93 YALE L.J. 362 (1983).

10. Id.

11. See e.g., *In re Quinlan,* 70 N.J. 10, 355 A. 2d 647, 664 (1976).

12. See e.g., *Lane v. Candura,* 6 Mass. App. 377, 376 N.E. 2d 1232 (1978); *Matter of Quackenbush,* 156 N.J. Super. 282, 383 A. 2d 785 (1978).

13. See e.g., *Custody of a Minor,* 383 Mass. 697, 434 N.E. 2d 601, 604–605, 607 n. 9 (1982); *In re Dinnerstein,* 6 Mass. App. 466, 380 N.E. 2d 134, 135–36 (1978); *Brophy v. New Eng. Sinai Hosp.,* 398 Mass. 417 (1986).

For some groups of chronically ill, the right to refuse treatment ought to be offered as an option from the inception of treatment, itself. Knowing of this option would be particularly re-assuring for the unsophisticated who might be unaware of it. Appelbaum & Roth, Patients Who Refuse Treatment in Medical Hospitals, 250 J.A.M.A. 1296 (1983).

14. Report of the Clinical Care Committee of the Massachusetts General Hospital, Optimum Care for Hopelessly Ill Patients, 295 NEW ENG. J. MED. 362 (Aug. 12, 1976).

15. Smith, *Triage:* Endgame Realities, 1 J. CONTEMP. HEALTH L. & POL'Y 143 (1985).

16. Report of the Clinical Care Committee of the Massachusetts General Hospital, Optimum Care for Hopelessly Ill Patients, 295 NEW ENG. J. MED. 362 (Aug. 12, 1976).

17. Id.

18. "Do Not Resuscitate Orders: The Proposed Legislation and Report of the New York State Task Force on Life and the Law" (1986).

See generally, Mooney, Deciding Not to Resuscitate Hospital Patients: Medical and Legal Perspectives, 1986 Ill. L. Rev. 1025.

19. The Proposed Legislation, "Orders Not to Resuscitate," numbers twelve actual pages in the Report, itself at 59–71.

Governor Mario Cuomo signed into law, on August 7, 1987, Chapter 818 of the Laws of New York, that adopted in major part the findings and legislative proposals of this Report. It became effective April 1, 1988, and was codified as N.Y. Pub. Health Law § § 2960–2978 (McKinney 1987).

For a comparison of the new law with the proposals of the New York State Task Force on Life and the Law, see Comment, Do Not Resuscitate Orders: A Matter of Life or Death in New York, 4 J. Contemp. Health L. & Pol'y (1988).

20. §§2(6), 3, 4. N.Y. Pub. Health Law § 2962 (McKinney 1987). This secondary cite to McKinney is the correlative citation to the Task Force Proposal. Both citations will be presented in footnotes 20–46. Hereinafter, the New York Health Law Code citation will be McKinney § _____.

21. Id. at §5. McKinney § 2964.

22. Id. at §4. McKinney § 2964 (2)(a)(b).

23. Id. at §5. McKinney § 2964.

24. Id. McKinney § 2964 (2)(b).

25. Id. at §5(3). McKinney § 2964 (3).

26. Id.

27. Id. at §§3, 4, 5. McKinney § 2962 (1).

28. Id. at §5. See McKinney § 2961 (3).

29. Id. at §6. McKinney § 2965.

30. Id. McKinney § 2965 (2), (3).

31. Id. Id.

32. Id. McKinney § 2965 (5)(c).

33. Id. at §6(5). McKinney § 2965 (5)(a).

34. Id. at §7. McKinney § 2966 (1).

35. Id. at §8. McKinney § 2967 (2)(a).

36. Id. Id.

37. Id. at §9. McKinney § 2968.

38. Id. at §10. McKinney § 2969 (1).

39. Id. McKinney § 2969 (2).

40. Id. McKinney § 2969 (3).

41. Id. at §13. See McKinney § 2972.

42. Id. at §14. McKinney § 2973 (1).

43. Id. at §14(2). McKinney § 2973 (3).

44. Id. at §15. McKinney § 2974.

45. Id. Id.

46. Id. at §16. McKinney § 2975.

47. Younger, Do-Not-Resuscitate Orders: No Longer Secret, But Still a Problem, HASTINGS CENTER RPT. 24, 32 (1987).

48. Id. at 33.

49. Malcolm, Reassessing Care of Dying: Policy Seen Evolving from A.M.A. Opinion, N.Y. TIMES, Mar. 17, 1986, at 1, col. 1.

50. Capron, Legal and Ethical Problems in Decisions for Death, 14 LAW, MED. & HEALTH CARE 141 (Sept. 1986).

51. Id.

52. Supra note 49.

53. TIME Mag., Mar. 31, 1986, at 60.

See Cohn, Doctor and Patient, Facing Death Together, Wash. Post Health Mag., Mar. 15, 1988, at 14, col. 1.

54. Am. Medical News, Nov. 28, 1986, at 13, col. 1.

55. Id.

56. Id.

57. See TIME Mag., Mar. 31, 1986, at 60; supra note 49.

58. Id.

Previously, the AMA had acknowledged that, "When a terminally ill patient's coma is beyond doubt irreversible and there are adequate safeguards to confirm the accuracy of the diagnosis, all means of life support may be discontinued, "but also acknowledged that most patients of this nature were probably given basic measures such as hygiene and artificial nutrition," 1982 A.M.A.'s Judicial Council, CURRENT OPINIONS, A.M.A. 9–10 (1982), as reported in, President's Commission for the Study of Ethical Problems in Medicine and Biomedical and Behavioral Research, DECIDING TO FOREGO LIFE-SUSTAINING TREATMENT: ETHICAL, MEDICAL, AND LEGAL ISSUES IN TREATMENT DECISIONS at 186, 187 (1983).

See Colburn, Withholding Food, Wash. Post Health Mag., Jan. 26, 1988, at 15, col. 1.

59. President's Commission for the Study of Ethical Problems in Medicine and Biomedical and Behavioral Research, DECIDING TO FOREGO LIFE-SUSTAINING TREATMENT: ETHICAL, MEDICAL, AND LEGAL ISSUES IN TREATMENT DECISIONS at 90, 288 (1983).

See also, Lynn & Childress, Must Patients Always be Given Food and Water?, 13 HASTINGS CENTER RPT. 17, 20 (1983).

60. Annas, Do Feeding Tubes Have More Rights than Patients, 16 HASTINGS CENTER RPT. 16 (1986).

61. Colburn, AMA Ethics Panel Revises Rules on Withholding Food, WASH. POST HEALTH MAG., April 2, 1986, at 9.

62. 70 N.J. 10, 355 A.2d 647, *cert. denied sub nom., Garger v. New Jersey,* 429 U.S. 922 (1976).

63. Id.

64. Supra note 60.

65. TIME Mag., Mar. 31, 1986, at 60.

See, Somerville, 'Should the Grandparents Die?' Allocation of Medical Resources with an Aging Population, 14 LAW, MEDICINE & HEALTH CARE 158 (Sept. 1986).

66. Id.

67. Id.

68. Supra note 61.

69. Id.

70. Id.

71. Statement of the Council on Ethical and Judicial Affairs, Am. Med. Assoc., March 15, 1986, "Withholding or Withdrawing Life Prolonging Medical Treatment."

72. Id.

73. Id.

74. Id.

75. Doctor Sees Trend Not to Resuscitate, WASH. POST, June 13, 1982, at A1, col. 3.

76. Brown & Thompson, Nontreatment of Fever in Extended-Care Facilities, 300 NEW ENG. J. MED. 1246 (May 31, 1979).

77. Id.

78. Id.

79. D. CRANE, THE SANCTITY OF SOCIAL LIFE: PHYSICIAN'S TREATMENT OF CRITICALLY ILL PATIENTS 58–61 (1975); Noyes, Jochimsen & Travis, The Changing Attitudes of Physicians Toward Prolonging Life, 25 J. AM. GERIATRIC SOC. 470 (1977).

80. Weiner, New VA Policy Allows Right-to-Die Instructions, WASH. POST, Sept. 20, 1983, at 1, col. 1.

81. Id.

82. Id.

83. Id.
See generally, Kuhse, The Case for Active Voluntary Euthanasia, 14 LAW, MEDICINE & HEALTH CARE 125 (Sept. 1986).

84. Cohen, Ethical Problems of Intensive Care, 47 ANESTHESIOLOGY 217 (1977).

85. McCormick, To Save or Let Die and the Dilemma of Modern Medicine in HOW BRAVE A NEW WORLD 339 at 349 (R. McCORMICK ed. 1981).

86. Supra notes 71–74.

87. Supra note 80.

88. Supra note 79.

89. Fletcher, Love is The Only Measure, 83 COMMONWEALTH 427 (1966).

90. See G. SMITH, GENETICS, ETHICS AND THE LAW 2, 8, 164 (1983).

91. DECIDING TO FOREGO LIFE–SUSTAINING TREATMENT: A REPORT ON THE ETHICAL, MEDICAL AND LEGAL ISSUES IN TREATMENT DECISIONS 288 (1983).

92. TIME Mag., Mar. 31, 1986, at 60.

93. Paris & McCormick, The Catholic Tradition on the Use of Nutrition and Fluids, AMERICA 356, 358 (May 2, 1987).

94. Id.

95. Id. at 361.
See generally, D. KELLY, THE EMERGENCE OF ROMAN CATHOLIC MEDICAL ETHICS IN NORTH AMERICA (1979).

96. Gostin, The Right to Choose Death: The Judicial Trilogy of Brophy, Bouvia, and Conroy, 14 LAW, MED. & HEALTH CARE 198, 201 (Sept. 1986).

97. Id. at 200.

98. Id.

99. Childress, When is it Morally Justifiable to Discontinue Medical Nutrition and Hydration? in BY NO EXTRAORDINARY MEANS at 81 (J. LYNN ed. 1986).

100. Id. at 81.

See Hilfiker, Allowing the Debilitated to Die: Facing Ethical Choices, 308 NEW ENG. J. MED. 716 (1983).

101. Supra note 96 at 201.

102. Id.

103. Id. at 201.

104. Williamson, Prolongation of Life or Prolonging the Act of Dying? 202 J.A.M.A. 162 (1967).

105. *Guidelines,* ps. 46–52.

106. Id. at 35–42.

107. Id. at 43–56.

108. Id. at 57–62.

109. Id. at 63–68.

110. Id. at 69–75.

111. Id. at 6–8.

112. Id. at 119–125.

113. Id. at 122.

114. D. CALLAHAN, SETTING LIMITS: MEDICAL GOALS IN AN AGING SOCIETY 140 (1987).

115. Id. at 143.

116. Id. at 198, 199.

117. Id. at 181, 182.

118. Id. at 190.

For individuals declared to be *brain dead,* no further care of any kind (medical or nursing) is directed; for the *severely demented* it is held to be inappropriate to terminate nursing care or nutrition and hydration either artificial *or* natural; for those suffering a *mild impairment of competence* advanced life supports are not morally required; for the *severely ill, mentally alert patient,* nursing care should be provided and for the *physically frail, mentally alert* patient, extended intensive care and advanced life supports are unwarranted at public expense. Id. at 182–183.

119. Id. at 187, 191.

120. Id. at 188.

121. Id. at 196.

122. Id.

123. 50 Fed. Register. 14873 (1985). Child Abuse Amendments of 1984, Pub. L. No. 98-457, 98 Stat. 1749, 42 U.S.C. §701 *passim.*

124. Id.

125. See generally Smith, Quality of Life, Sanctity of Creation: Palliative or Aptheosis? 63 NEB. L. REV. 709 (1984): H. KUHSE, P. SINGER, SHOULD THE BABY LIVE (1986).

126. Moskop & Saldanha, The Baby Doe Rule: Still a Threat, HASTINGS CENTER RPT. 8, 9 (April 1986).

127. Id. at 14.

128. Id.

129. See Donley, A Brave New World of Health Care, 2 J. CONTEMP. HEALTH L. & POL'Y 47, 51 (1986); Pellegrino, Rationing Health Care: The Ethics of Medical Gatekeeping, 2 J. COMTEMP. HEALTH L. & POL'Y 23 (1986); Smith, Death Be Not Proud: Medical, Ethical and Legal Dilemmas in Resource Allocation: 3 J. CONTEMP. HEALTH L. & POL'Y 47 (1987).

Admitting the strong inference from the literature that the terminally ill receive proportionately more expensive treatment than do other patients, and that—consequently—the issue of extended care should be made within the reasonable context of cost containment, a distinguished group of researchers has set three basic goals for cost containment policies for the terminally ill: develop more reasonable criteria for the admission of patients to intensive or critical care units; promote the autonomy of patients and their families as decision makers in health care issues of this nature and, further, develop and thereby promote alternative forms of institutional care such as the hospice. Bayer, Callahan, Fletcher, et al, The Case of the Terminally Ill: Morality and Economics, 309 NEW ENG. J. MED. 1490, 1491, 1493 (1983).

See also, Fries, Aging, Natural Death and the Compression of Morbidity, 303 NEW ENG. J. MED. 130, 131, 135 (1980). It is predicted that the mean average age at death by the year 2009 will be 82.4 years. Id. at 131.

130. See, The President's Commission for the Study of Ethical Problems in Medicine and Biomedical and Behavioral Research, DECIDING TO FOREGO LIFE-SUSTAINING TREATMENT: ETHICAL, MEDICAL AND LEGAL ISSUES IN TREATMENT DECISIONS at 5, n. 3, 228.

See also, Englehardt, Ethical Issues in Aiding the Death of Young Children in BENEFICENT EUTHANASIA at 180, 187 (M. KOHL ed. 1975) where he proposed a concept of injury for continuance of existence as an analogue of the concept of the tort of wrongful life. "It seems reasonable . . . that the life of children with diseases that involve pain and no hope of survival should not be prolonged. Id. at 189.

See generally, R. WEIR, SELECTIVE NON TREATMENT OF HANDI-CAPPED NEWBORNS (1984).

131. Survey, Euthanasia: Criminal, Tort, Constitutional and Legislative Considerations, 48 NOTRE DAME L. REV. 1202, 1203 (1973); Cantor, Conroy: Best Interests, and the Handling of Dying Patients, 37 RUTGERS L. REV. 543, 549 (1985).

132. Clarke, The Choice to Refuse or Withhold Medical Treatment: The Emerging Technological and Medical-Ethical Consensus, 13 CREIGHTON L. REV. 813, 815 (1980).

133. See e.g., *In re President & Directors of Georgetown College, Inc.,* 331 F. 2d, 1000, 1009 (D.C. Cir. 1964), *reh. en banc denied,* 331 F. 2d 1010 (D.C. 1964); *John F. Kennedy Memorial Hosp. v. Hestor,* 58 N.J. 576, 279 A. 2d 670, 674 (1971).

134. See e.g., *In re Conroy,* 98 N.J. 321, 351, 486 A. 2d 1209, 1224 (1985); *Satz v. Perlmutter,* 362 So. 2d 160, 162 (Ct. App. Fla. 1978).

135. See e.g., *In re* Melidio, 88 Misc. 2d 974, 390 N.Y.S. 2d 524 (Sup. Ct. 1976).

136. 4 ENCYCLOPEDIA OF BIOETHICS 1502 (W. REICH ed. 1976).

137. Byrn, Compulsory Lifesaving Treatment for the Competent Adult, 44 FORD-HAM L. REV. 1, 35 *passim* (1975).

138. See *Jacobson v. Massachusetts*, 197 U.S. 11 (1905), the leading case where state interest — in preventing the spread of smallpox — was held to supersede the right of a person to refuse treatment innoculation. See generally, G. GRIEZ, J. BOYLE, JR., LIFE AND DEATH WITH LIBERTY AND JUSTICE (1977).

139. *Bartling v. Superior Court (Glendale Adventist Medical Center)*, 163 Cal. App. 2d 186, 196, 209 Cal. Rptr. 220, 225 (1984).

140. *Satz v. Perlmutter*, 362 So. 2d 160, 162 (Fla. Dist. Ct. App.), *aff'd*, 379 So. 2d 359 (Fla. 1980). See also, *Superintendent of Belchertown State School v. Saikewicz*, 373 Mass. 728, 370 N.E. 2d 417 (1977); *In re Quinlan*, 70 N.J. 10, 355 A. 2d 647, *cert. denied* 429 U.S. 922 (1976); *In re Colyer*, 99 Wash. 2d 114, 660 P. 2d 738 (1983).

141. *In re Quinlan*, 70 N.J. 10, 23–29, 355 A. 2d 647, 655–657, *cert. denied* 429 U.S. 922 (1976); *Superintendent of Belchertown State School v. Saikewicz*, 373 Mass. 728, 737–740, 370 N.E. 2d 417, 423–424 (1977); *Eichner v. Dillon*, 72 A.D. 2d 431, 468–469, 426 N.U.S. 2d 517, 545 (1980) *modified sub. nom.*, *In re* Storar, 52 N.Y. 2d 363, 420 N.E. 2d 64, 438 N.Y.S. 2d 266 (1981).

142. *In re Quackenbush*, 156 N.J. Super. 282, 290, 383 A. 2d 785 (Morris County Ct. 1978); *John F. Kennedy Memorial Hosp. v. Heston*, 58 N.J. 576, 279 A. 2d 670 (1971).

143. P. RAMSEY, ETHICS AT THE EDGES OF LIFE: MEDICAL AND LEGAL INTERSECTIONS 1–14 (1978).

144. Sherlock, For Everything There is a Season: The Right to Die in the United States, 1982 BRIGHAM YOUNG UNIV. L. REV. 545, 560 (1982).

While, in itself, the principle of beneficence could arguably support a course of medical treatment against the wishes of a patient, it is restricted or conditioned by the principles of respect for persons or recognition, simply, of one's autonomy. This principle of personal respect mandates full attention be given to the competency of the patient who disclaims the use of prolongation of life-sustaining therapies. J. CHILDRESS, WHO SHOULD DECIDE? PATERNALISM IN HEALTH CARE 175 (1982).

145. Comment, Balancing the Right to Die with Competing Interests: A Socio-Legal Enigma, 13 PEPPERDINE L. REV. 109 (1985).

146. Id. at 127, 128.

For example, a patient might be classified as terminal because it is expected that he will live for nine months even though there are other significant variables: his treatment may be intrusive and painful and he has expressed a desire to be removed from life-sustaining mechanisms in order his certain death in a more dignified manner. Another case might find a patient with a more terminal condition in that he has but a five-month life expectancy and his treatment is less intrusive and thus less painful and, furthermore, his desire to be taken off life-supporting treatment has wavered. Here, the condition of the patient would have to be more serious in order to meet or overcome the competing state interest in preserving life. Id. A set of additional interesting hypotheticals are posed at 125 *passim*.

147. R. VEATCH, DEATH, DYING AND THE BIOLOGICAL REVOLUTION 146 (1976).

148. J. NOWAK, R. ROTUNDA, J. YOUNG, CONSTITUTIONAL LAW 764 (2d ed. 1983).

149. Id.

150. See e.g., *In re Conroy*, 98 N.J. 321, 486 A. 2d 1209, (1985); *Bartling v. Superior Court*, 163 Cal. App. 2d 186, 209 Cal. Rptr. 220 (1984).

151. See Jonas, The Right to Die, HASTINGS CENTER RPT. 31 (1978).

152. See e.g., *In re Conroy*, 98 N.J. 321, 348; 486 A. 2d 1209, 1222 (1985); *Bartling v. Superior Court*, 163 Cal. App. 2d 186, 195, 209 Cal. Rptr. 220, 225 (1984); *In re Colyer*, 99 Wash. 2d 114, 132–33, 660 P. 2d 738 (1983); *In re Storar*. 52 N.Y. 2d 363, 420 N.E. 2d 266, 276, *cert. denied*, 454 U.S. 858 (1981).

153. *Bartling v. Superior Court*, supra; *In re Storar*, supra; *In re Quinlan*, 70 N.J. 10, 40, 355 A. 2d 647, 663, *cert. denied*, 429 U.S. 922 (1976); *Superintendent of Belchertown State School v. Saikewicz*, 373 Mass. 728, 370 N.E. 2d 417, 425–427 (1977); *Matter of Spring*, 380 Mass. 629, 405 N.E. 2d 115 (1980).

The Court in *In re Yetter* held, "... . the right of privacy includes a right to die with which the State should not interfere where there are no minor or unborn children and no clear and present danger to public health, welfare or morals." 62 Pa. D. & C. 619, 623 (1973).

See also, G. GRIEZ, J. BOYCE, JR., LIFE AND DEATH WITHOUT LIBERTY AND JUSTICE 98 *passim* (1977); Delgado, Euthanasia Reconsidered — The Choice of Death as an Aspect of the Right of Privacy, 17 ARIZ. L. REV. 474 (1975).

154. See e.g., *In re Osborne*, 294 A. 2d 372 (D.C. 1972); *In re Estate of Brooks*, 32 Ill. 2d 361, 205 N.E. 2d 435 (1965).

See generally, Ford, Refusal of Blood Transfusions by Jehovah Witnesses, 10 CATH. LAW. 212 (1964); Paris, Compulsory Medical Treatment and Religious Freedom: Whose Law Shall Prevail? 10 U. SAN F. L. Rev. 25 (1975).

155. See e.g., *In the Matter of the Guardianship of Joseph Hamlin, an Incompetent Person*, 102 Wash. 2d 810, 689 P. 2d 1372 (1984).

156. Friendly, The Courts and Social Policy: Substance and Procedure, 33 U. MIAMI L. REV. 21 (1978).

157. See *Truman v. Thomas*, 27 Cal. 3d 285, 611 P. 2d 902, 165 Cal. Rptr. 308 (1980); *Crisher v. Spak*, 122 Misc. 2d 355, 471 N.Y.S. 2d 741 (1983).

158. *In re Conroy*, 98 N.J. 321, 486 A. 2d 1209 (1985).

159. 70 N.J. 10, 355 A. 2d 647 (1976).

160. Id.

See also, Hirsch & Donovan, The Right to Die: Medico-Legal Implications of In re Quinlan, 30 RUTGERS L. REV. 267 (1977).

161. 70 N.J. 10, 51–52, 355 A. 2d 647, 669–70 (1978).

162. 381 U.S. 479 (1961).

163. Id.

164. Quinlan Dies — Decade in Coma, USA TODAY, June 12, 1985 at 1A, col. 2.

165. 373 Mass. 728, 370 N.E. 2d 417 (1977).

166. Id. at 733, 370 N.E. 2d 421.

167. Id. at 739, 370 N.E. 2d at 424.

The recognition of the right to refuse medical treatment in appropriate circumstances "must extend to the case of an incompetent, as well as a competent, patient because the value of human dignity extends to both." Id. at 427.

168. Curran, The Saikewicz Decision, 298 NEW ENG. J. MED. 499 (1978).

169. 373 Mass. 728, 752–73, 370 N.E. 2d 417, 431 (1977).

170. 370 N.E. 2d at 423.

Distinguishing its course of action here from that taken in *Quinlan* by the New Jersey Supreme Court, where a parental determination was made that, drawing from past experiences with Ms. Quinlan, she would not have wished respiratory assistance, the *Saikewicz* court had no such interested relative who could advise it regarding what Mr. Saikewicz would have wished proposed — and thus the court was compelled to intervene. Id. at 430.

171. 373 Mass. at 741, 370 N.E. 2d at 425.

172. 373 Mass. at 731, 732, 370 N.E. 2d at 420–422.

173. Id.

174. Id.

The two powerful principles for which the *Saikewicz* court stood were that courts, not physicians, should make the ultimate decisions about life and death and that these judicial decisions should always reflect what the patient, himself, would have chosen. Stone, Judges As Medical Decision Makers, 12 THE HUMAN LIFE REV. 84, 91 (1986).

175. In re Dinnerstein, 1978 Mass. App. Adv. Sh. 736, 380 N.E. 2d 134 (1978).

176. Id.

177. 380 N.E. 2d 134, 139 (1978).

178. 380 N.E. 2d at 139.

179. *In re Spring,* 80 Mass. Adv. Sh. 1209, 405 N.E. 2d 115 (1980).

180. Id. at 1210, 405 N.E. 2d at 117.

181. Id. at 1212, 405 N.E. 2d at 118.

182. Id.

183. 405 N.E. 2d at 123.

184. Id.

185. 405 N.E. 2d at 117, 122.

186. 405 N.E. 2d at 122.

187. 73 A. D. 2d 431, 426 N.Y. 2d 517 (App. Div. 1980), *rev'd. sub nom., In re Storar,* 52 N.Y. 2d 363, 438 N.Y.S. 2d 266 (1981).

188. Id.

189. *In re Eichner,* 52 N.Y. 2d 363, 377, 438 N.Y.S. 2d 266, 276.

190. Id. at 378, 438 N.Y.S. 2d at 273–274.

191. *In re Storar,* 52 N.Y. 2d 363, at 380, 438 N.Y.S. 2d 274, 275.

192. 438 N.Y.S. 2d at 269.

193. 426 N.Y.S. 2d at 537–41.

194. 52 N.Y. 2d 363 at 378, 438 N.Y.S. 2d at 273–74.

195. 52 N.Y. 2d 363, 438 N.Y.S. 2d 266 (1981).

196. Id. at 374–75, 438 N.Y.S. 2d at 271–272.

197. Id. at 380, 438 N.Y.S. 2d at 275.

198. *In re Eichner,* 52 N.Y. 2d 363 at 382-382, 438 N.Y.S. 2d at 276.
199. 147 Cal. App. 2d 1006, 195 Cal. Rptr. 484 (1983).
200. 195 Cal. Rptr. at 490.
201. Id. at 491.
202. Id.
203. Id.
204. Id. at 491, 492.
205. Id. at 491.
206. Id. at 486.
207. Id.
208. Id.
209. Id. at 490.
210. Id.
211. Id. at 491.
212. Id.
213. Id. at 493.
214. Id.
   The factors to be considered here would include relief of suffering, preservation or restoration of functioning capacities, quality and extent of sustainable "life," and the impact of the ultimate decision on those closest to the patient. Id.
   See also, Lo, The Death of Clarence Herbert: Withdrawing Care is Not Murder, 101 ANNALS OF INT. MED. 248 (1984); Lynn & Childress, Must Patients Always Be Given Given Food and Water? HASTINGS CENTER RPT. 17 (1983).
   The Massachusetts Court of Appeal cited approvingly to *Barber* in the case of *In the Matter of Mary Hier,* 18 Mass. App. Ct. 200, 464 N.E. 2d 959 (1984) as support for its ruling that a ninety-two year old incompetent patient who had pulled out her gastrostomy tube, need not undergo a forced surgical intervention in order to have the tube reinserted. Id. at 201. The decision of the court was made with full knowledge of the fact that the patient's intravenous feeding was used as but a short-term technique for maintaining hydration rather than a balanced diet. Id. at 203. Acknowledging that the substituted judgment test was valid and proper as was used here (Id. 207, 209, 210), the court concluded medical nutrition and fluids were to be administered as with any other medical intervention: in accordance with a balancing of the benefits and the burdens to the patient (Id. at 207) and that such actions do not in certain circumstances violate either the law or medical ethical. Id.
215. *Bartling v. Superior Court of Los Angeles County,* 163 Cal. App. 3d 186, 209 Cal. Rptr. 220, 221 (1984).
216. Id.
217. Id.
218. 209 Cal. Rptr. at 222.
219. Id.
220. Id.
221. Id.
222. Id. at 223.
223. Id. at 224, 225.

224. Id. at 225.
225. Id. at 226, citing approvingly to *Superintendent of Belchertown v. Saikewicz.*
226. 209 Cal. Rptr. at 226.
227. Id.
228. Id. at 224.
    See, *In re Torres,* 357 N.W. 2d 332 (Minn. 1984). See also *Kenneth Foody v. Manchester Memorial Hospital,* 40 Conn. Supp. 127, 482 A. 2d 713 (Conn. Sup. Ct. 1984); *Rasmussen v. Fleming,* 154 Ariz. 207, 741 P.2d 674 (1987).
229. *In re Conroy,* 98 N.J. 321, 486 A. 2d 1209 (1985).
230. Id. at 338–39, 486 A. 2d at 1217–18.
231. Id.
232. Id.
233. Id.
234. *In re Conroy,* 188 N.J. Super. 523, 529–30, 457 A. 2d 1232, 1236 (Ch. Div. 1983).
235. *In re Conroy,* 190 N. J. Super. 453 at 461, 464 A. 2d 303 at 306–07 (App. Div. 1983).
236. Id. at 475, 464 A. 2d at 315.
237. Id. at 469–70, 464 A. 2d at 312.
238. Id.
239. 190 N. J. Super. at 466, 464 A. 2d at 312.
240. 98 N. J. 321 at 388, 486 A. 2d 1209 at 1244.
    The New York Court of Appeals determined that a nasogastric tube could not be withheld from an incompetent patient unless the patient—while competent—made a clear, resolute decision to reject such treatment. Matter of O'Connor, 57 U.S.L. Week 2241 (Oct. 14, 1988).
241. Id. at 361, 486 A. 2d at 1229.
242. Id. at 365, 486 A. 2d at 1232.
243. Id. at 366–67, 486 A. 2d at 1232.
244. Id. at 344–346, 486 A. 2d at 1240–1242.
245. Id.
246. Id.
247. For example, if the guardian of an incompetent believed under one of the objective tests that actions that would terminate life-sustaining treatments were in the patient's best interest and proceeded to follow the set procedure mandated by the court, treatment could be continued as a consequence of but one dissent from a family member. And, if the same judicially designed procedure were followed and a concurrence given by the patient's entire family that such actions were in the best interests of the patient, and assuming further all other conditions were satisfied, one of the two physicians necessarily appointed by the State Ombudsman for the Institutionalized Elderly—if hesitant to agree regarding the condition of the patient—could cause treatment to be continued. In a word, there are too many check-points that cause road-blocks mandated by the Conroy procedures. Case Comment, Natural Death: An Alternative in New Jersey, 73 GEO. L. J. 1331, 1351 (1985).
    See Annas, When Procedures Limit Rights: From Quinlan to Conroy, HASTINGS CENTER RPT. 24 (1985).

248. In the Matter of Nancy Ellen Jobes, 210 N.J. Super. 543, 510 A. 2d 133 (1986).

249. 510 A. 2d 133 at 134.

250. 510 A. 2d at 135. (Emphasis provided.)

In a landmark position taken by the State Attorney General of Maryland, it was held that where a physician has documented a patient, or his authorized surrogate's refusal of artificially administered sustenance, such action must be respected and is not in contravention of federal and state regulations requiring hospitals and nursing homes to meet the nutritional needs of their patients. Op. 88-046, in 73 Opinions of the Atty. General (1988).

251. Id.

252. 108 N.J. 394, 529 A.2d 434 (1987).

The United States District Court of Rhode Island ruled — in what appears to be the very first federal court decision on the issue — that the right of privacy (implicit in the 14th Amendment's Due Process Clause) encompasses the right to decline life sustaining medical treatment (e.g., nutrition and hydration). Here, the husband of a woman in a persistent vegetative state, sought the removal of her feeding tube. It was conceded that the patient, if competent, would have authorized removal of the tube. Gray v. Romeo, 57 U.S.L. Week 2256 (Nov. 1, 1988).

253. Id.

254. Id.

255. Id.

256. Id.

257. Id.

The Supreme Court of Missouri held on November 16, 1988, that where an incompetent has no hope of recovery from a persistent vegetative state — but is neither legally dead nor terminally ill — the state's interest in the preservation of life outweighs the patient's right to live and, thus, a guardian may not order a cessation of nutrition and hydration. Cruzan v. Harmon, 57 U.S.L. Week 2324 (Dec. 6, 1988).

258. Id.

259. Id.

260. Id.

261. Id.

262. Id.

263. Id.

Two other cases involving the right to refuse medical treatment were decided by the New Jersey Supreme Court with *Jobes* on June 24, 1987: *In re Farrell,* 108 N.J. 335, 529 A.2d 404 (1987) and *In re Peter,* 108 N.J. 365, 529 A.2d 419 (1987). Both cases underscore the right of self-determination in health care decision making.

264. 373 Mass. 728, 370 N.E. 2d 417 (1977).

265. 98 N.J. 321, 486 A.2d 1209 (1985).

266. See Sullivan, Jersey Judge Permits Denial of Food to Patient in Coma, N.Y. TIMES, April 24, 1986, at 17, col. 5.

See John F. Kennedy Memorial Hospital v. Bludworth, 452 So. 2d 921 (Fla. 1984) where a court refused to involve itself in determining whether a withdrawal of a respirator should be allowed — deferring instead to either the family or appointed guardian to discharge the incompetent's right to refuse extraordinary medical treatment.

267. 98 N. J. 321, 486 A. 2d 1209, 1237 *passim* (1985).

268. Supra, note 266.

In the *Jobes* case, there was convincing evidence that Mrs. Jobes had expressed, on previous occasions, her wish never to be sustained on artificial life supports if she became helpless. Id.

269. *Bouvia v. County of Riverside,* No. 159780, Sup. Ct. Riverside Co., Cal. Dec. 16, 1983, TR. 1238–1250.

270. *Bouvia v. Superior Court of Los Angeles County,* 179 Cal. App. 3d 1127, 225 Cal. Rptr. 297 (1986).

271. The trial court decision is reproduced in 1 ISSUES LAW & MED. 486 (1986) and references thereto are from this reproduction.

272. Id. at 486.

273. Id.

274. Id. at 487.

275. Id. at 491.

276. Id.

277. Id. at 489.

278. Id. at 487.

279. Id. at 488.

280. Id. at 490.

281. Van den Haag, A Right to Die? NAT'L REVIEW 45, 46 (May 9, 1984).

282. Annas, When Suicide Prevention Becomes Brutality: The Case of Elizabeth Bouvia, HASTINGS CENTER RPT. 20, 21 (1984).

283. Id. at 46.

284. Id.

285. Id.

See generally, Note, The Role of Law in Suicide Prevention: Beyond Civil Commitment — A Bystander Duty to Report Suicide Threats?, 39 STAN. L. REV. 929 (1987).

286. Bouvia v. Superior Court of Los Angeles County, 179 Cal. App. 3d 1127, 225 Cal. Rptr. 297 (1986).

See also, Annas, Elizabeth Bouvia: Whose Space Is It Anyway?, HASTINGS CENTER RPT. 24 (1986); Williams, The Right to Die, 134 NEW LAW JOURNAL 73 (1984).

287. Id.

288. *Bouvia v. Superior Court of Los Angeles County,* 179 Cal. App. 3d 1127, 225 Cal. Rptr. 297 at 302 (1986) citing to *Bartling v. Superior Court,* 163 Cal. App. 3d 186, 209 Cal. Rptr. 220.

289. 225 Cal. Rptr. at 301, citing to *Bartling v. Superior Court,* 163 Cal. App. 3d 186, 209 Cal. Rptr. 220.

290. 225 Cal. Rptr. at 300.

291. Id. at 304.

292. Id. at 306.

293. Id. at 303.

294. Id. at 305.

295. Id.

296. Id. at 306.

297. Id.

298. *In re Joseph G.,* 34 Cal. 2d 429, 194 Cal. Rptr. 163, 667 P. 2d 1176 (1983).

299. 225 Cal. Rptr. at 306.

In the case of *In re Requena,* 213 N.J. Super. 443, 517 A. 2d 869 (1986), the court compelled St. Clare's Riverside Medical Center, a Catholic-affiliated hospital, to allow the petitioner to remain as a patient, dying of amyotrophic lateral sclerosis ("Lou Gehrig's Disease), and—furthermore—to co-operate with her refusal of tubal feeding. This was ordered despite a contrary institutional policy against such procedures and the availability of another facility for her transfer. The court maintained that hospital staff sensibilities were subordinate to the psychological pain and trauma the transfer of the dying patient would bring to the patient, herself.

300. *Brophy v. New England Saint Hosp., Inc.,* 398 Mass. 417, 497 N.E. 2d 626, 628, 629 (1986).

301. Id.

302. Id

303. 497 N.E. 2d at 629–636.

304. Id. at 633.

305. Id. at 633, 634, 635.

306. See e.g., *Superintendent of Belchertown State School v. Saikewicz,* 373 Mass. 728, 370 N.E. 2d 417 (1977); *Matter of Spring,* 8 Mass. App. 831, 399 N.E. 2d 493 (1979); *Matter of Spring,* 300 Mass. 629, 405 N.E. 2d 115 (1980); *Matter of Dinnerstein,* 6 Mass. App. Ct. 466, 380 N.E. 2d 134 (1978); *Bouvia v. Superior Court for Los Angeles County,* 179 Cal. App. 3d 1127, 225 Cal. Rptr. 297 (1987).

307. 497 N.E. 2d at 635.

308. Id. at 637.

309. Id.

The trial court accepted evidence that showed the longest recorded survival by such means was thirty-seven years. Id.

310. Id. at 639.

311. Id.

312. 373 Mass. 728, 370 N.E. 2d (1977).

313. 497 N.E. 2d at 639.

314. Id. at 639, 640.

315. Id. at 636.

316. Id. at 637, 638.

317. See also *Corbett v. D'Alessandro.* 487 So. 2d 368 (Fla. Dist. Ct. App. 1986).

The Washington State Supreme Court held December 10, 1987, that a twenty-two year old woman suffering from Batten's disease (a terminal genetic, neurological condition)—though *not* comatose—but suffering severe and permanent mental deterioration, has a right under Washington law to have life-sustaining treatment withheld; here, specifically nasogastric tubes and intravenous feeding at her mother's request. *In re Grant,* 109 Wash. 2d 545, 747 P.2d 445 (1987).

318. *Brophy,* held particularly that acts of refusing medical treatment merely allow the particular disease to take its natural course and when death occurs eventually, it is the primary result of the underlying disease and not of self-inflicted injuries. Id. at 638. See also, *Rasmussen v. Fleming,* 154 Ariz. 200, 741 P.2d 667 (1987).

319. See Annas, Do Feeding Tubes Have More Rights Than People?, 16 HASTINGS CENTER RPT. 26 (1986); Gostin, A Right to Choose Death: The Judicial Trilogy of *Brophy, Bouvia,* and *Conroy,* 14 LAW, SCIENCE & MED. 198 (1986).

See also, Reidinger, Trends in the Law: Go Gentle into That Good Night — More States Recognize Right to Die, 74 A.B.A.J. 122 (1988).

On January 31, 1989, the Supreme Court of Connecticut held that the state Removal of Life Support System legislation authorizes the removal from a terminally ill patient of artificial life supports such as a gastrostomy tube. *McConnell v. Beverly Enterprises — Connecticut Inc.,* 209 Conn. 692 (1989).

320. Gostin, supra at 319.

321. *In re Conroy,* 98 N.J. 321, 486 A. 2d 1209, 1223 (1986).

322. Gostin, supra note 319 at 198.

323. Id.

See also, Annas, Fashion and Freedom: When Artificial Feeding Should be Withdrawn, 75 AM. J. PUB. HEALTH 685 (1985).

See generally, Wolhander, Voluntary Active Euthanasia for the Terminally Ill and the Constitutional Right of Privacy, 69 CORNELL L. REV. 363 (1984).

Chapter VI

A CONSTRUCT FOR DECISION MAKING

THE STRUCTURAL GOALS AND PROCEDURES

Because of the lack of uniformity and great variation in the factual situations of each case of critical and terminal illness, no one approach or procedural scheme is either possible or desirable; for the individual situation gives rise to and, indeed, mandates a functional or situational ethic of response.[1] Yet, certain goals can be set. While an advance directive requesting treatment should serve as an obvious guide for subsequent cases when it becomes necessary or operative, the management of a patient's actual case must be made in light of all current circumstances that may not have been foreseen by the patient, himself, when making his original directive.[2] When no medical alternative can be found to be acceptable to all concerned parties, a compromise should be sought.[3] If an institutional ethics committee exists, the compromise should be worked out there.[4] If the committee or some other type of intra-institutional review mechanism is unable to find a consensus solution or compromise, and disagreement continues between at least two of either the health care professionals, or members of the family, then legal redress should be sought in the courts.[5]

It is urged strongly that the courts avoid making decisions among several treating options—and, instead, seek the appointment of a responsible surrogate decision maker or guardian who in turn is charged with collecting and considering relevant information, making a decision regarding the course that should be effected and thereupon reporting it to the court.[6] It is, in the long run, more promotive of the justice of each case if the duly appointed surrogate is given wide discretion in his decision making authority; for *routine* resort to the judicial process should never be encouraged by legislatures or invited by the courts themselves.[7] Expeditious and sensitive decision making is more obtainable through intra-institutional processes than protracted judicial inquiry.[8] Ethical and social policy frameworks can also more easily take form through the

deliberative processes of committee work that in turn can be of incalcu-
lable value for future similarly related cases.[9] The well-being of the
patient remains the focus and primary goal of all decision making for the
incapacitated,[10] while, for the competent, an unyielding recognition of
his right to pursue rational and self-enlightening acts of self-determination
should be guaranteed.

THE FAMILY

The extent of the right of the family as a unit to direct or, for that
matter, interfere with treatment or non-treatment decisions of the competent or incompetent terminally ill *or* non-terminal family member or
with a court appointed guardian or other surrogate decision maker,
remains an unsettled area of contention. While the right of assertion by
the family of its self-determination in the areas of tragic choice being
considered here cannot remain unfettered and unchallenged, intrusions
by the state or primary health care providers should be limited generally
to those cases where the limits of reason and the best interests of the
incapacitated family member are being disregarded in a flagrant manner.[11]

In countering the point of familial autonomy or merely expanding
upon the circumstances where a parent or family member should not be
regarded as having sole decision making authority over issues of withholding or withdrawing life-sustaining treatments, three situations can
be submitted where intrusion or challenge must be made: when the
parent or other family member is unable to comprehend the relevant
medical facts of the instant case; when they are emotionally unstable and
when they appear to be placing their own interests before those of the
severely handicapped or at-risk family member.[12] Indeed, physicians are
often the much better qualified surrogate decision maker than a parent or
other family member—this being the case simply because of their greater
objectivity, technical knowledge and expertise and professional involvement with similarly patterned illnesses or complex health problems.[13]

Once a decision is made to provide life-sustaining treatment for a
seriously ill patient, the issue of the costs of that continuing care come
into focus.[14] Families need programs that can support their valiant efforts
here—especially so when special care is required either at home or in the
institutions for care of the severely handicapped infant or terminally ill
adult.[15] Hospice care is becoming a more viable option for the last stages
of a terminal illness and, thus, a way in which specialized care can be

given within a family-like setting, but without the physical and economic drain of at-home care.[16]

REASONABLENESS

Social justice demands that each individual be given an equal opportunity to maximize his individual potential. Yet, points are often reached in the lives of individuals where their maintenance is a defiance of the basic concept of both humanitarianism and social justice. When an individual's condition represents a negation of "truly human" qualities or a "relational potential," then the best form of treatment should be no treatment at all.[17] State otherwise, when—regardless of age—therapies would be futile and thus run counter to the best interests of a patient, then they should not be undertaken.[18] Thus, efficacious treatment may be no treatment. Although the standard of potentiality for human relationships does not admit of absolute precision, in the case for example of an anencephalic infant born without a brain, or a patient who has been declared brain dead, it is rather obvious that these individuals would not qualify for developing the potentiality.[19]

In less clearly defined cases, one would expect to find the standard of reasonableness—that is always flexible and responsive to individual factual applications—to be a useful if not dominant construct for decision making. Thus, admixed and balanced with or against reasonableness would be specific social policies emerging from each particular case, together with the principle of justice and humaneness or love.[20] Determination of the best interests of one family member would of necessity be based upon individual family beliefs in a set of social and spiritual values as well as economic ones. If an act renders more harm than good to the at-risk individual, and to those around him, the act would be viewed properly as unloving, unjust or inhumane. The concepts of ordinary and extraordinary treatment in essence, then, are little more than value judgments that determine whether a given course of treatment poses an undue hardship on the patient or provides some hope for a direct benefit.[21]

The crucial point of understanding is that in determining whether to allow a terminally ill competent individual, an incompetent one, or one such as Elizabeth Bouvia who is not terminal but is in a state of physical degeneration and incapacity that pain remains a constant given in her life so long as she lives, the lynch-pin to any course of reasonable action is but a basic cost/benefit analysis. Its stated simplicity belies its complexity in application but, as a construct, reasonableness will always be incapable of absolute pre-determination; for its application will always be set in motion and constrained by the dynamics of each specific case and the accepted standards of medical science and practice.

INTRA-INSTITUTIONAL REVIEW

Hospital ethics committees are, of course, immensely valuable as a construct for decision making. Yet, it is not considered cost-effective to convene the committee for every ethical problem that presents a difficulty —only when "the ethical deliberations reveal an exceedingly complex question does the entire committee become involved."[22]

Perhaps even more crucial to validating decisions regarding the withholding or withdrawal of life-sustaining treatment than an ethics committee is a prognosis committee; for if there is unanimity in this regard, the work of any other committee is minimized greatly. Thus, when a disagreement arises between a personal physician and the family over the diagnosis and prognosis for an at-risk patient family member or between a court appointed guardian when no family exists, the matter should be referred to a prognosis committee within the treating institution, itself, for a second opinion. Maintained on an *ad hoc* basis and selected as need arises for each case on its own merit, the committee would be composed of the patient's physician and at least two other staff physicians. If a unanimous agreement were to be reached that there was no reasonable medical probability of a return by the handicapped patient to a rational or functioning state, then the prognosis would be entered in the patient's medical record.[23]

The only function, essentially, of such a committee would be to confirm the diagnosis and the prognosis. It would be this Committee's responsibility, and not that of a court, to determine when there was no longer any reasonable hope for recovery for the terminally ill patient.[24] If disagreement among the prognosis committee, itself, arose, then that matter would be then sent to a full multi-disciplinary ethics committee for hope-for resolution instead of judicial determination. Even if the ethics review committee were for some reason to take review of the case, with a unanimous prognosis committee opinion having been given already, it would be hoped that such thorough and professional "preliminary" work by the prognosis committee would make the work of the ethical reconsideration lightened considerably.

It has been suggested that the easiest way to avoid the cumbersome machinery of committee decision making would be simply to relieve the physician of responsibility—civil and criminal—for those actions which he might undertake in *good faith* to relieve a terminally ill person.[25] This standard of reasonableness, or good faith, is—as has been shown—a well tested and proven mechanism for assessing degrees of responsibility within the law. Although pre-eminently fair, the current disjointed state of legal, social and medical attitudes is such that a course of definite action of the nature proposed here, even though undertaken in good faith, would most surely subject the physician to professional censure as well as civil and criminal liability. To be sure, the directions are clear from a handful of cases and a significant legislative pattern among the states that terminating actions may be rendered by a physician acting in good faith *if* certain defined procedures (and approvals) are followed. But, swift preemptory, good faith actions of a unilateral order—lacking in an historical or evidentiary record of deliberation and consultation— have yet to be approved. Perhaps because of this state of affairs in the United States, the Dutch physicians who participate regularly in efforts to assist terminally ill patients with acts of enlightened self-determination or what is commonly termed voluntary active euthanasia, regularly employ—as has been observed—a "team" of doctors, nurses and a representative of the patient's faith or religion to counsel and evaluate the validity of requests made by terminally ill patients for relief. These teams also provide a level of protection and cover for the doctor's legal liability if he were ever to be prosecuted.[26] This team has an obvious parallel in the prognosis committee, or ethical review committee used in the United States. Of course the similarity in this procedural mechanism here between Holland and the United States is the only aspect of sharing —for the national attitude regarding the right of enlightened self-determination creates an altogether more tolerant and accepting attitude toward death by this means than is evident in the United States.

What of the non-terminal yet severely suffering patient who can expect little more than years of suffering, incapacitation and personal degradation because of his Elizabeth Bouvia type of condition? Surely, he should have the same rights of self-determination as other less-afflicted citizens. After a period of psychological counseling, the physically and mentally distressed individual should present his case to an ethical tribunal for the required permission and/or assistance in ending his life.[27] Composed of a wide sampling of independent individuals, representing legal, ethical, medical, social, religious and lay interests, the tribunal would be empowered—without interference, consultation or deference to any other interest group, family or otherwise—to decide the issue before it. Ideally, the contrary or opposing position to that taken by the petitioner would be presented by an *amicus curiae.* If the committee rules in favor of the petitioner, then he is to be assisted in ending his life. Contrariwise, if the committee rules against the petitioner, the deliberative issue is whether he should be involuntarily committed to a state or other proper institution and retained, and thereby prevented from seeking his goal.

If, after counseling for a reasonable period of time, and the individual still wishes to exercise his right of enlightened self-determination, should he be enabled by assistance? In other words, could he ask for another review by the same or another ethics committee or appeal to the courts to either assist him actively or allow him passively to exercise his right? It has been suggested that before consent should be given, the proper authorities should satisfy themselves that it is the "patient's firm and well considered choice and not the desperate whim of a mood of melancholia and not under pressure from others."[28] *Bouvia* does, however, present evidence of a possible wedge that may be developing that would recognize a right of rational self-determination regardless of whether the applicant or petitioner is terminal. Elizabeth Bouvia won the right not to be forced fed and to starve herself if she wished. By the court's reasoning, the doctors who of necessity will have to assist her in carrying out her wish (or right to refuse treatment) by maintaining her morphine pump and directing her nursing care are directing the execution of her constitutionally protected right—not assisting in her demise. If more courts were to see the simple validity of this position, the current state of confusion would be ended. This cannot be expected realistically, however, to come quickly because traditional values about the preservation of "life"—no matter within a degenerative state or not—dictate a response that curtails those who wish to act otherwise and label them as irrational in their thinking.

LEGISLATIVE AND JUDICIAL RESPONSES

Model laws, such as the Uniform Rights of the Terminally Ill and The Uniform Determination of Death Act, and enactments such as Natural Death Acts, Living Wills and Durable Powers of Attorney,[29] while certainly not complete guarantees of an individual's right, with ease, to control his final act of self-determination, are to be applauded for the constructive value they have in both setting a direction and, similarly, being responsive to a growing number within a contemporary society who demand of the government more and more an option to die with dignity. New laws need to be passed now correcting the practical difficulties that have been discussed previously, encountered in the administration of these legislative structures.[30]

If more and more enlightened courts of the caliber of *Barber*,[31] *Bartling*,[32] *Bouvia*,[33] and *Brophy*[34] can be found to assert, and to guarantee, the right of every citizen — competent or incompetent, terminal or nonterminal — to refuse life-sustaining treatments and to be assisted in the execution of this right without an imposition of civil or criminal liability as with Elizabeth Bouvia, the task of developing a firm judicial construct for decision making will be more attainable within a time frame heretofore thought almost impossible to meet within this century.

Ever faithful, or at least cognizant, of their role as interpreters of the law, however, and thus often reluctant to be bold, creative architects, the courts need strong and unequivocal legislation to assist them in their responsibility to interpret the law within a framework of contemporary values; legislation that has certain uniform characteristics that unerringly structure recognition of individual rights of autonomy, but also protect the vulnerable from exploitation.[35] More specifically, such legislative guarantees should assure that competent patients — or, those who not only can appreciate but understand the nature and consequences of their actions — have an unequivocal right to refuse any form of treatment, that would include artificial nutrition and hydration. Second, all citizens should be able to execute a document — as, for example a living will — that not only declares their wishes for the manner of care they are to receive would they become incompetent, but designate a surrogate decision maker to enforce these wishes through a durable power of attorney. Finally, in cases where a patient becomes incompetent and has neglected to make such a declaration or designation of one as his surrogate decision maker, the patient's legally appointed guardian should be able to direct that any medical treatment (including artificial feeding) be withheld or withdrawn. This course of action should be mandated upon the guardian's demonstration to the immediate health care providers that this action is what the patient would wish; or, that such a cause of action would be consistent with the patient's best interests by virtue of the fact that a simple cost-benefit analysis shows clearly that the burden met through the use of continued treatments "outweigh any reasonably hoped for benefits from the patient's perspective."[36]

OTHER PERSUASIVE GUIDELINES

The proposals of the New York State Task Force on Life and the Law for a model legislative scheme for providing clear guidelines for decision making for orders not to resuscitate are yet another positive step toward shaping a workable construct to aid health care providers, afflicted at-risk patients and surrogate decision makers with complete knowledge of their rights and responsibilities.[37] The proposals—many of which have been enacted into law—also add a degree of momentum to the growing legislative efforts to acknowledge the right of critically ill patients to assert their right of autonomy either during their competency or subsequent incompetency and, at the same time, act as a spur for other state legislative initiatives in this specific area.

Opinions by the American Medical Association's Council on Ethical and Judicial Affairs for establishing Guidelines for Withholding or Withdrawing Life Prolonging Medical Treatment for Terminally Ill or Irreversibly Comatose Patients and recognizing the ethical propriety for withdrawing life-sustaining medical treatment, including food and water,[38] afford the physicians and other health care providers with a professional endorsement of actions of this nature.

Protocols such as the 1976 one by the Massachusetts General Hospital on Optimum Care for Hopelessly Ill Patients,[39] also aid in the development of a workable standard of good medical practice (or reasonableness) in rendering assistance to the terminally ill.

Finally, the framework for principled decision making—as it continues to draw upon these and other yet to be realized constructs in this critical area of concern—can be but strengthened by a record that discloses few legal prosecutions have been sustained for aiding, abetting or assisting one in an act of suicidal self-destruction,[40] and that the growing trend is to adhere to the same prosecutorial standard of legal inaction for passive euthanasia.[41]

Taken as a unit, these various constructs show that there is, indeed, a developing framework for principled medical, legal, ethical, philosophical, religious and economic decision making; not perhaps as clear and distinct as might be hoped for, but unmistakenly there for use and application.

Whether they are recognized for their value or taken as obstructions to the principle of sanctity and preservation of life depends, ultimately, on the attitude of the participants in each particular critical intervention. Perhaps, with time, they will be viewed correctly as but keys to humane or reasonable value judgments.

CONCLUSIONS

Whether the acceptance of a policy of rational suicide opens "the floodgate to genocide and eliminating people who are feebleminded,"[42] and "introduces a bias in favor of death"[43] thereby allowing suicide to be viewed as "socially useful"[44] or opens the door and finds a crowd eager to enter the passageway,[45] is pure speculation. The fear of the "slippery slope" has accompanied every new release of knowledge—scientific or otherwise.[46] Such fears discount the rationality of man and demean his ability to meet and resolve personal crises. Indeed, the humanistic essence and postivism of all religious and theological thinking is also largely discounted by expression of such meddlesome fears.

Perhaps the only permissible restraints—temporal or physical—that can justifiably be placed on a suicidal person are those productive either of the goal of autonomy or rational liberty.[47] John Stuart Mill, in his essay "On Liberty," states unequivocally that the only purpose for which power can be exercised over any member of society is to prevent harm to others; protecting for one's own good—either physical or moral—is not a sufficient warrant for intrusion.[48] Why should not a sane person decide his own fate—if it is a rational choice—and not based on impulse or impelled by emotion? Is there some broader societal or moral interest in compelling life for those who would commit suicide?

The judiciary has—when forced to enter the forum of critical decision making—begun to elucidate criteria from which a construct for principled decision making may be undertaken. No sweeping generalizations, but carefully crafted standards designed for subsequent percental value emerge as guidelines to provide a developing pathway for the all too many similar case determinations that follow. Although death with dignity may not be acknowledged uniformly by all states to be a fundamental right, it is at least being recognized more and more as a humane and enlightened policy.

To bemoan what has been occurring with the courts as a triumph of the functional ethics prescription for death—"death by neglect, dehydration and starvation" for the incurably disabled and then conclude dramatically that "the protection afforded life and equality" by the Constitution has been discarded for the hopefully suffering and terminally ill,[49] is to display an illogical and pro-life blindness that subscribes to the shiboleth that where there is breath, there is "life." It is also a position that fails *totally* to attempt to appreciate or understand the eloquent balancing test of individual costs versus societal benefits used in determining the course of action (or inaction) to be administered in each, individual problem of terminal illness. Determining a patient's best interests are thus grounded in policies of reasonableness and humaneness. It is an inhumane and calloused type of argument that directs the agony of death be protracted by the use of gastronomy tubes, nasogastric tubes and other means of providing aliementation under the guise of being efficacious treatment and proceeds to wrap itself in a distorted manner with the pro-life anti-abortion movement.

Suicide. Euthanasia. Rational Suicide. Assisted Rational Suicide. Beneficent Euthanasia. Are these words and theories soon to be of the past? Hopefully so. What has been proposed could, rightly, be thought of as being somewhat revolutionary. But, in contempory times, sometimes revolutions are necessary in order to correct situations that are seemingly incorrectable by no other means. Perhaps, if a responsive judiciary and astute state legislature continue at their current pace, declaring one's inherent right of enlightened self-determination, be he competent or incompetent, incapacitated or not, to determine the nature and form of this last rite of passage, no dramatic revolution in taxonomy will be necessary. Perhaps the revolution will come from *within* the system, itself, and thereby give rise to a new socio-legal-medical and cultural appreciation of death and the dying process as humane and—when possible—non-violent. And, an attitude that will recognize old age not as a terminal disease, yet not a stage in the life cycle mandating that all means should be employed to maintain, and thus disenfranchise,[50] all terminally ill or otherwise incapacitated individuals. If this attitude were to be developed, it then might follow that whether a right to decline life-sustaining treatment is to be regarded as a right to commit suicide (assisted or autonomous) and effect euthanasia, as well, becomes moot. For, inherent to the attitude, itself, would be an acceptance that, in whatever context of self-determination the central issue is cast or the dilemma seen, a moral and a legal right would indeed be bestowed upon the individual to act—for whatever enlightened or rational purposes he wishes—to end his life by refusing life-sustaining medical treatment.[51]

ENDNOTES

1. President's Commission for The Study of Ethical Problems in Medicine and Biomedical and Behavioral Research: A Report on the Ethical, Medical and Legal Issues in Treatment Decisions—DECIDING TO FOREGO LIFE–SUSTAINING TREATMENT at 192 (1983).

2. Id. at 193.

3. Id.

4. Id. at 194.

5. Id. at 194, 154.

6. Id.

7. Id. at 196, 156.

8. Supra note 1 at 169.

9. Id. at 161.

10. Id. at 170.

11. McCormick, To Save or Let Die: The Dilemma of Modern Medicine in HOW BRAVE A NEW WORLD at 339, 378 (R. McCORMICK ed. 1981).

See generally, Smith, Defective Newborns and Government Intermeddling, 25 MED. SCI. & L. 44 (1985).

12. R. WEIR, SELECTIVE NON–TREATMENT OF HANDICAPPED NEW-BORNS 269 (1984).

13. Id.

14. Supra note 1 at 228.

15. Id.

16. See S. LACK, R. BUCKINGHAM, FIRST AMERICAN HOSPICE (1978); S. STODDARD, THE HOSPICE MOVEMENT (1978); Note, Hospice: The Legal Ramifications of a Place to Die, 56 IND. L. J. 673 (1981).

17. Supra note 11 at 349.

18. Supra note 1 at 6.

19. See generally, Fletcher, Indicators of Humanhood, 13 HASTINGS CENTER RPT. 1 (1972).

20. Fletcher, Love is the Only Measure, 83 COMMONWEALTH 427 (1966).

21. R. McCormick, NOTES ON MORAL THEOLOGY 1965 THROUGH 1980, at 565 (1981).

See generally, Annas, Toward an Ethic of Ambiguity, HASTINGS CENTER RPT. 25 (1984).

22. Purtilo, Ethics Consultations in the Hospital, 311 NEW ENG. J. MED. 983, 984 (1984).

See generally, Newman, Treatment Refusals for the Critically and Terminally Ill: Proposed Rules for The Family, The Physicians and The State, 3 N.Y.L. SCH. HUMAN RIGHTS ANN. 35, 80–81 (1985).

23. *In re Colyer,* 99 Wash. 2d 114, 134–35, 660 P. 2d 738, 749–50 (1983).

24. Id. at 135, 660 P. 2d at 750.

25. G. WILLIAMS, THE SANCTITY OF LIFE AND THE CRIMINAL LAW, Ch. 8 at 340 (1958).

26. Appleyard, The Last Appointment, THE SUNDAY TIMES MAG. (London), June 7, 1987, at 13.

27. See generally, Dagi, The Ethical Tribunal in Medicine in 1 ETHICAL, LEGAL AND SOCIAL CHALLENGES TO A BRAVE NEW WORLD at 201 (G. SMITH ed. 1982).

28. A. TOYNBEE, MAN'S CONCERN WITH DEATH 158 (1968). See also, M. HEIFETZ, THE RIGHT TO DIE 97–98 (1975).

29. Supra Ch. III, notes 24–36.

30. Id.

31. 147 Cal. App. 3d 1006, 195 Cal. Rptr. 484 (1983).

32. 163 Cal. App. 3d 186, 209 Cal. Rptr. 200 (1984).

33. 179 Cal. App. 3d 1127, 225 Cal. Rptr. 297 (1986).

34. 398 Mass. 417, 497 N.E. 2d 626 (1986).

35. Annas, Fashion and Freedom: When Artificial Feeding Should be Withdrawn, 75 AM. J. PUB. HEALTH 685, 688 (1985).

36. Id.

37. Do Not Resuscitate Orders: The Proposed Legislation and Report of the New York Task Force on Life and the Law (1986).

38. See TIME Mag., Mar. 31, 1986, at 60.

39. Report of the Clinical Care Committee of the Massachusetts General Hospital, Optimum Care for Hopelessly Ill Patients, 295 NEW ENG. J. MED. 362 (Aug. 12, 1976).

40. See 66 A.B.A.J. 1499, 1501 (1980); Survey, Euthanasia: Criminal, Tort, Constitutional and Legislative Considerations, 48 NOTRE DAME L. REV. 1202, 1206 (1973).

See also, Engelhardt & Malloy, Suicide and Assisting Suicide: A Critique of Legal Sanctions, 36 So. W.L.J. 1003, 1019, 1120 (1982).

41. Id.

42. 66 A.B.A.J. 1499, 1501 (1980).

43. TIME Mag., Mar. 21, 1983 at 85.

44. Id.

45. Barber, Guilty Verdict in Mercy Killing, USA TODAY, May 10, 1985, at 3A, col. 1.

46. Delgado & Miller, God, Galileo and Government: Toward Constitutional Protection for Scientific Inquiry in 1 ETHICAL, LEGAL AND SOCIAL CHALLENGES TO A BRAVE NEW WORLD 231 (G. SMITH ed. 1982).

47. Fromer, A Few Good Words for Suicide, WASH. POST, Sept. 6, 1981, at C1, col. 1.

48. The Six Great Humanistic Essays of John Stuart Mill, On Liberty, Ch. 1 Introduction at 135 (A. LEVI ed. 1969).

49. Destro, Quality-of-Life Ethics and Constitutional Jurisprudence: The Demise

of Natural Rights and Equal Protection for the Disabled and Incompetent, 2 J. CONTEMP. HEALTH L. & POL'Y 71, 121, 123 (1976).

50. See Jonas, The Right to Die, HASTINGS CENTER RPT. 31, 34 (Aug. 1978).

51. See, J. CHILDRESS, WHO SHOULD DECIDE? PATERNALISM IN HEALTH CARE 163 (1982).

AUTHOR INDEX

SUBJECT INDEX